ELSEVIER

Pocket Guide to

ONCOLOGY
DRUGS &
REGIMENS

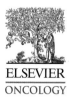

ELSEVIER
ONCOLOGY

www.oncologydrugguide.com

ELSEVIER ONCOLOGY
46 Green Street, 2nd floor
Huntington, NY 11743

PRESIDENT AND PUBLISHER:
Anthony J. Cutrone

Production Director: Wendy McGullam

Editorial Manager: Gail M. VanKoot

Senior Editors: Randi Londer Gould, Conor Lynch

Design Director: Edwin S. Geffner

Consultant: John A. Gentile, Jr.

Director, Sales and Marketing: Joseph T. Schuldner

Group Sales Director: Timothy Wolfinger

National Sales Representative: David Horowitz

Sales Administrator: Devin Gregorie

PROJECT DIRECTED AND MANAGED BY MEDVANTAGE PUBLISHING

Director: Patricia Dwyer Schull, RN, MSN

Clinical Manager: Minnie Bowen Rose, BSN, MEd

Editorial Manager: Karen C. Comerford

Design Manager: Stephanie Peters

Website Development Manager: Joseph J. Clark

Research Coordinator and Analyst: Lois Piano, RN, MSN, EdD

Clinical Editors: Julie M. Gerhart, MS, RPh; Cheryl A. Grandinetti, PharmD; Cynthia Saver, RN, MS

Editors: Naina Chohan, Kathy E. Goldberg, Andy McPhee, Doris Weinstock

Designers: Joseph J. Clark, Jan Greenberg

Editorial Assistant: Julia S. Knipe

Cover Design: John Hubbard

ISBN-1-4160-3422-6

Copyright © 2006 Elsevier, Inc. All rights reserved. No part of this publication may be reproduced, stored in a retrieval system, or transmitted in any form or by any means (electronic or mechanical, photocopying, recording, or otherwise) without prior written permission from the publisher (except for brief quotations in critical articles and reviews). Printed in the United States of America.

For information, contact Elsevier Oncology at address above or call (631) 424 8900.

The authors and publisher have made every effort to ensure that the information in this book is accurate and in accord with the standards accepted at the time of publication. However, pharmacology is a constantly changing field; as new research and clinical experience broaden knowledge, changes in treatment and drug therapy may become appropriate or necessary. Readers are urged to check the most current product information provided by the manufacturer of each drug they administer or dispense to verify the recommended dosage, administration method, duration of therapy, and contraindications. It is the responsibility of the licensed prescriber, relying on experience and knowledge of the patient, to determine dosages and the optimal treatment for each individual patient. Also, standard safety precautions must be followed. Neither the author nor publisher assumes any liability for any injury and/or damage to persons or property arising from this publication.

Visit our website at:
www.oncologydrugguide.com.

Table of contents

Advisors and contributors

Advisors

Martin Abeloff, MD
Professor and Chair
Department of Oncology
Director, Sidney Kimmel Comprehensive Cancer Center at Johns Hopkins
Baltimore, Md.

David Henry, MD
Vice Chairman, Department of Medicine
Clinical Professor of Medicine
Joan Karnell Cancer Center at Pennsylvania Hospital
Philadelphia, Pa.

Maurie Markman, MD
Vice President for Clinical Research
MD Anderson Cancer Center
University of Texas
Houston

William McGivney, PhD
Chief Executive Officer
National Comprehensive Cancer Network
Jenkintown, Pa.

Christine Miaskowski, RN, PhD, FAAN
Professor and Chair
Department of Physiological Nursing
University of San Francisco
San Francisco, Calif.

Steven Rosen, MD
Director
Robert H. Lurie Comprehensive Cancer Center of Northwestern University
Chicago, Ill.

Neal Slatkin, MD, DABPM
Director
Department of Supportive Care, Pain, and Palliative Medicine
City of Hope National Medical Center
Duarte, Calif.

Contributors

Helena Joy Altizer, RN, BSN, OCN
Kootenai Medical Center
North Idaho College
Coeur d'Alene, Idaho

Lisa M. Barbarotta, RN, MSN
Oncology Nurse
Hospital of St. Raphael's
New Haven, Conn.

Ronald H. Blum, MD
Professor, Department of Medicine
Albert Einstein College of Medicine
Director, Cancer Center
Beth Israel Medical Center
New York, N.Y.

Joseph Bubalo, PharmD, BCPS, BCOP
Assistant Professor of Medicine
Oregon Health and Science University Hospital & Clinics
Portland, Ore.

Katherine L. Byar, MSN, APRN, BC
Hematological Malignancy Nurse Practitioner
University of Nebraska Medical Center
Omaha, Nebr.

Joanna E. Cain, RN, BSN
President
Auctorial Pursuits, Inc.
Wilmington, N.C.

Gregory T. Clark, BS, BCOP
Clinical Oncology Pharmacist
Rochester General Hospital
Rochester, N.Y.

Julene A. Diedrich, RN, APNP, OCN
Nurse Practioner,
Oncology/Hematology
Marshfield Clinic
Marshfield, Wis.

Robert Dreicer, MD, FACP
Professor of Medicine
Cleveland Clinic Lerner College of Medicine
Director Genitourinary Medical Oncology
Taussig Cancer Center
Cleveland Clinic Foundation
Cleveland, Ohio

Matthew E. Eckley, PharmD
Clinical Pharmacy Specialist—Oncology
Huntsville Hospital
Huntsville, Ala.

Karen M. Fancher, PharmD, BCOP
Clinical Pharmacist
Blood & Marrow Transplantation
H. Lee Moffitt Cancer Center & Research Institute
Tampa, Fla.

Julie M. Gerhart, MS, RPh
Manager, Pharmacy Affairs
Merck & Co., Inc.
West Point, Pa.

Dawn Goetz, PharmD, BCOP
Clinical Pharmacist
Medical Oncology
H. Lee Moffitt Cancer Center and Research Institute
Tampa, Fla.

Janet Gordils-Perez, RN, MA, OCN, APN-C
Advance Practice Nurse
Cancer Institute of New Jersey
New Brunswick, N.J.

Cheryl A. Grandinetti, PharmD
Senior Clinical Research Pharmacist
Cancer Therapy Evaluation Program
Division of Cancer Treatment and Diagnosis
National Cancer Institute
Rockville, Md.

Myke Green, PharmD, BCOP
Clinical Oncology Pharmacist
H. Lee Moffitt Cancer Center and
    Research Institute
Tampa, Fla.

Karen Groth, MSN, CNS, ARNP
Cancer Care Northwest
Spokane, Wash.

**Heidi D. Gunderson, PharmD,
    BCOP**
Hematology/Oncology
    Pharmacist
Mayo Clinic
Rochester, Minn.

David H. Henry, MD
Vice Chairman, Department of
    Medicine
Clinical Professor of Medicine
Joan Karnell Cancer Center at
    Pennsylvania Hospital
Philadelphia, Pa.

**John E. Loughner, PharmD,
    BCOP**
Supervisor, Oncology Pharmacy
Strong Memorial Hospital
Rochester, N.Y.

**Ellyn E. Matthews, RN, PhD,
    AOCN, CRNI**
Assistant Professor
University of Colorado at Denver
    and Health Sciences Center
Denver, Colo.

Mary Jane McDevitt, RN, BS
Case Manager
Home Care
Delaware County Memorial
    Hospital
Drexel Hill, PA

MaryJo Moran, RPh, BCOP
Clinical Pharmacist
Park Ridge Hospital
Rochester, N.Y.

Jose R. Murillo, Jr., BS, PharmD
Clinical Specialist II—
    Hematology/Oncology
The Methodist Hospital
Houston, Tex.

**Cindy L. O'Bryant, PharmD,
    BCOP**
Assistant Professor
University of Colorado at Denver
    and Health Sciences Center
School of Pharmacy
Denver, Colo.

Christopher L. Olek, RPh, BCOP
Oncology Pharmacist
Strong Memorial Hospital
Rochester, N.Y.

**Joanna Maudlin Pangilinan,
    PharmD, BCOP**
Pharmacist
University of Michigan Health
    System
and
Cascade Hemophilia Consortium
Ann Arbor, Mich.

Vivian Park, PharmD, BCOP
Clinical Coordinator
Division of Pharmacy Services
Memorial Sloan-Kettering Cancer
Center
New York, N.Y.

**Martha Polovich, RN, MN,
AOCN**
Oncology Clinical Nurse
Specialist
Southern Regional Medical
Center
Riverdale, Ga.

Martha Purrier, RN, MN, AOCN
Oncology Clinical Nurse
Specialist
Manager, Inpatient Oncology
Unit
Virginia Mason Medical Center
Seattle, Wash.

Michele Riccardi, PharmD
Pharmacy Clinical Coordinator
Midstate Medical Center
Meriden, Conn.

Mujahid A. Rizvi, MD, MPH
Fellow, Division of Hematology/
Oncology
Northwestern University
Chicago, Ill.

Cynthia Saver, RN, MS
President
CLS Development, Inc.
Columbia, Md.

**Nancy Thompson, RN, MS,
AOCNS**
Clinical Nurse Specialist
Swedish Cancer Institute
Seattle, Wash.

**John P. Timoney, PharmD,
BCOP**
Clinical Pharmacy Specialist
Memorial Sloan-Kettering Cancer
Center
New York, N.Y.

**Gene A. Wetzstein, PharmD,
BCOP**
Clinical Specialist, Hematology
H. Lee Moffitt Cancer Center and
Research Institute
Tampa, Fla.

**Robert C. Wolf, PharmD, BCPS,
BCOP**
Pharmacotherapy Coordinator—
Hematology/Oncology
Assistant Professor Mayo Clinic
College of Medicine
Mayo Clinic
Rochester, Minn.

Daisy Yang, PharmD, BCOP
Clinical Pharmacy Specialist
MD Anderson Cancer Center
University of Texas
Houston, Tex.

User's guide

Over the last 30 years, we have witnessed substantial progress against cancer. Advances in biomedical knowledge continue to enhance our understanding of the causes and mechanisms of the disease. For some types of cancer, such advances have permitted earlier cancer detection and diagnosis and have led to more effective treatments.

In addition, newly identified molecular targets are transforming the way oncology drugs are developed and used. Today, rational drug combinations are used not just to treat cancer but also to cure some cancers that once proved uniformly fatal. Such combinations also have helped prevent relapse and improve the quality of life in patients with certain cancers.

Responding to practitioners' needs

As we move closer toward the ultimate goal of curing and eliminating cancer, oncology practitioners face the ever-escalating challenge of keeping up with the rapid pace of developments. Staying abreast of ongoing discoveries and advances is critical for professionals who prescribe or dispense oncology drugs or provide care for cancer patients.

To keep your pharmacologic knowledge base up-to-date, you must have a ready source of current, reliable, and accurate dosage information as well as the most important prescribing considerations at your fingertips. The *Elsevier Pocket Guide to Oncology Drugs & Regimens* was created to serve this vital purpose.

How to use this book

This book has two main sections, plus appendices that address important topics in oncology practice.

Drug monographs

The first section offers condensed monographs for the most important and most commonly used chemotherapy drugs. Monographs are arranged alphabetically by generic drug name. In each monograph, information appears in the order shown below.

• **Generic name:** Generic drug name(s) in the United States, along with salts and other variant names when applicable. If the drug label includes an FDA-assigned "black box" warning, a special logo (⊠) appears next to the generic name.

- **Trade name** (when applicable)**:** All trade, or brand, names available in the United States
- **Indications and dosages:** FDA-approved indications and dosages, followed (when applicable) by selected off-label uses. Only those indications relevant to oncology or supportive care are listed. Where appropriate, pediatric dosages are given separately.
- **Special considerations:** Important information on dosage modification, preparation and administration, and patient monitoring. If the drug poses a risk to healthcare workers who handle, prepare, or administer it, a special icon (⧗) appears.

Regimens

The second section of the book presents the most commonly used chemotherapy regimens (both single- and combination-agent regimens), shown alphabetically by cancer-specific disease type. For each regimen, you'll find information on supportive therapy that the regimen may necessitate.

Appendices

Appendices cover important topics in oncology practice, including:
- common abbreviations
- formulas for calculating body surface area
- supportive therapy for adverse reactions to chemotherapy or the disease process, with guidelines to help you assess and manage such problems as nausea and vomiting, anemia, neutropenia, diarrhea, and stomatitis
- hazardous drug management, including preparation and administration guidelines for hazardous parenteral, oral, and noninjectable drugs.

For a complete list of references to the information included in this pocket guide, see "References" on www.oncologydrugguide.com. For more comprehensive information on the drugs included in this pocket guide, see its companion product, *The Elsevier Guide to Oncology Drugs & Regimens.* You are also urged to check the most current product information provided by the manufacturer of each drug.

Elsevier's oncology drug information program

The Elsevier Pocket Guide to Oncology Drugs & Regimens is one of four integrated components of a unique, multidimensional oncology drug information program created after extensive research on the information needs of practicing oncology physicians and nurses. Other components include *The Elsevier Guide to Oncology Drugs & Regimens*, its PDA version, and the companion website, www.oncologydrugguide.com.

Dedicated to improving cancer care

Elsevier Oncology is dedicated to improving cancer care by providing up-to-date information and educational resources to healthcare professionals and patients in the fight against cancer. For practitioners who prescribe, dispense, or administer oncology drugs, *The Elsevier Pocket Guide to Oncology Drugs & Regimens* puts crucial drug facts at your fingertips.

Anthony J. Cutrone
President and Publisher
Elsevier Oncology

abarelix ⊠
Plenaxis

Indications and dosages
➥ Palliative treatment of advanced symptomatic prostate cancer when luteinizing hormone–releasing hormone agonist therapy is inappropriate or surgical castration has been refused and one or more of the following exists: risk of neurologic compromise due to metastases, ureteral or bladder outlet obstruction due to local encroachment or metastatic disease, or severe bone pain from skeletal metastases persisting despite opioid analgesia

Adults: 100 mg I.M. into gluteal muscle on days 1, 15, and 29, and every 4 weeks thereafter

Special considerations
• Only physicians enrolled in Plenaxis PLUS (Plenaxis User Safety) Program may prescribe drug.
• Obtain serum transaminase levels before starting drug and periodically thereafter.
• Before reconstituting, gently shake vial. Hold at 45-degree angle and tap lightly on table to break up caking.
• Reconstitute one vial (113 mg) with 2.2 ml normal saline injection for single I.M. injection.
• Give entire reconstituted suspension I.M. immediately.
• For at least 30 minutes after each injection, watch for allergic reaction.
• Monitor patient response by measuring total serum testosterone level before administration on day 29 and every 8 weeks thereafter.
• Periodic serum prostate-specific antigen measurement may also be considered.

aldesleukin ⊠
Proleukin

Indications and dosages
➥ Metastatic renal cell carcinoma
Adults: 600,000 international units/kg by I.V. infusion over 15 minutes every 8 hours for maximum of 14 doses. After 9-day rest, repeat sched-

▶▶ Potentially carcinogenic

ule for another 14 doses, to maximum of 28 doses per course, as tolerated.

➥ Metastatic melanoma

Adults: 600,000 international units/kg by I.V. infusion over 15 minutes every 8 hours for maximum of 14 doses. After 9-day rest, repeat schedule for another 14 doses, to maximum of 28 doses per course, as tolerated.

Off-label uses (selected)

➥ Malignant melanoma
➥ Non-Hodgkin's lymphoma

Special considerations

• Follow hazardous drug guidelines for preparation and administration.
• Drug may cause capillary leak syndrome (CLS).
• Withhold drug in patients with reduced organ perfusion. Recovery from CLS begins shortly after drug is discontinued.
• Discontinue drug if moderate to severe lethargy or somnolence develops.
• Restrict therapy to patients with normal cardiac and pulmonary function.
• Reconstitute with 1.2 ml sterile water for injection. Swirl but do not shake vial. After reconstitution, each ml contains 18 million units (1.1 mg/ml).
• Dilute reconstituted drug in 50 ml D_5W and infuse over 15 minutes.
• Watch for delayed adverse reactions.
• Monitor patient for irritability, confusion, and depression, which may indicate bacteremia or early bacterial sepsis, hypoperfusion, occult CNS cancer, or direct drug-induced CNS toxicity. Drug-induced mental status changes may progress for several days before recovery begins.
• Decreased neutrophil function may lead to infection and delayed healing.
• Watch for unexplained weight changes, hypotension, chest pain, heart murmurs, palpitations, irregular pulse, dyspnea or other respiratory impairment, and abnormal bleeding.
• Monitor kidney and liver function test results frequently.
• Monitor patient for pulmonary infiltration, which may appear by day 4 of therapy and usually resolves within a few weeks after drug is stopped.

☒ FDA black-box warning

- Evaluate patient for vision problems shortly after start of therapy.
- Watch for dermatologic effects, including skin peeling, angioedema, urticaria, and erythema nodosum.

---

alemtuzumab ⊠
Campath

Indications and dosages
➡ B-cell chronic lymphocytic leukemia in patients treated with alkylating agents who failed fludarabine therapy
Adults: 3 mg subcutaneously (commonly used but not FDA-approved route) daily or as 2-hour I.V. infusion daily. When tolerated, increase to 10 mg. When tolerated, initiate maintenance dosage of 30 mg/day three times a week on alternate days for up to 12 weeks. Dosage escalation takes 1 to 2 weeks.

Special considerations
- Follow hazardous drug guidelines for preparation and administration.
- Stop therapy during serious infection, serious hematologic toxicity, or other serious toxicity until event resolves.
- Stop therapy permanently if autoimmune anemia or thrombocytopenia occurs.
- Obtain baseline CBC with differential and platelet count.
- Do not administer by I.V. bolus or push.
- For I.V. infusion, dilute in 100 ml normal saline solution or D_5W and infuse over 2 hours.
- Administer diphenhydramine and acetaminophen, as indicated, 30 minutes before infusion to decrease risk of serious adverse reactions.
- Evaluate for hypotension during infusion.
- Monitor patient weekly for anemia, neutropenia, and thrombocytopenia (platelet count below 50,000/mm³).
- Evaluate CD4+ count after treatment until it recovers to 200 cells/mm³ or more.
- Take precautions against excessive bleeding and use extreme caution during invasive procedures.

---

altretamine ⊠
Hexalen

Indications and dosages
➡ Palliative treatment of persistent or recurrent ovarian cancer after cisplatin or alkylating agent–based combination therapy
Adults: 260 mg/m² P.O. daily in four divided doses for either 14 or 21 consecutive days in 28-day cycle

OFF-LABEL USES (SELECTED)
➡ Small-cell lung carcinoma

Special considerations
• Follow hazardous drug guidelines for preparation and administration.
• Temporarily discontinue (for 14 days or longer) and subsequently restart at 200 mg/m² daily if GI intolerance does not improve with symptomatic measures, WBC count is below 2,000/mm³, granulocyte count is below 1,000/mm³, platelet count is below 75,000/mm³, or progressive neurotoxicity occurs.
• If neurologic symptoms fail to stabilize on reduced dosage schedule, discontinue drug indefinitely.
• Evaluate peripheral blood counts before each course.
• Give an antiemetic before administration to help control nausea and vomiting.
• Give after meals or at bedtime to help prevent adverse reactions.
• Monitor hematocrit, hemoglobin, platelet count, and WBC count with differential at least monthly, before each course, and as clinically indicated.

amifostine
Ethyol

Indications and dosages
➡ Reduction of incidence of moderate to severe xerostomia in patients undergoing postoperative radiation treatment for head and neck cancer
Adults: 200 mg/m² I.V. once daily, infused over 3 minutes, starting 15 to

30 minutes before standard fraction radiation therapy (1.8 to 2 Gy)
➡ Reduction of cumulative renal toxicity caused by repeated cisplatin administration in patients with advanced ovarian cancer or non-small-cell lung cancer

Adults: 910 mg/m^2 I.V. once daily infused over 15 minutes, starting 30 minutes before chemotherapy. If full dose cannot be given, subsequent cycles should be administered at 740 mg/m^2.

OFF-LABEL USES (SELECTED)

➡ Myelodysplastic syndromes
➡ Protection against cisplatin- and paclitaxel-induced neurotoxicity
➡ Reduction of mucositis in patients receiving radiation therapy or radiation combined with chemotherapy

Special considerations

• Temporarily discontinue infusion if systolic blood pressure decreases.
• Give antiemetics, including I.V. dexamethasone and serotonin 5-HT$_3$ receptor antagonist, before and during amifostine administration.
• Interrupt antihypertensive therapy for 24 hours before amifostine administration.
• Administer as short-term I.V. infusion over 15 minutes; prolonged infusions increase risk of hypotension and vomiting.
• Monitor blood pressure every 5 minutes during infusion and thereafter as indicated.
• Monitor hydration status carefully, especially when giving drug with chemotherapy agents with high emetic risk, such as cisplatin.
• Continue to monitor blood pressure and hydration throughout therapy.

aminoglutethimide
Cytadren

Indications

OFF-LABEL USES (SELECTED)

➡ Metastatic prostate cancer
➡ Breast and prostatic carcinoma

⯮ Potentially carcinogenic

Special considerations
- Institute treatment in hospital until patient achieves stable dosage regimen.
- If rash persists beyond 8 days or becomes severe, discontinue drug. Restart at lower dosage after mild or moderate rash disappears.
- Monitor plasma cortisol and serum electrolyte levels and thyroid and liver function test results periodically.
- Adrenocortical hypofunction may occur, especially with stressful conditions.
- Drug may suppress adrenal aldosterone production and may cause orthostatic or persistent hypotension.

anastrozole
Arimidex

Indications and dosages
➡ Hormone-receptor-positive or hormone-receptor unknown locally advanced or metastatic breast cancer in postmenopausal women; advanced breast cancer in postmenopausal women with disease progression after tamoxifen therapy

Adults: 1 mg P.O. daily continued until tumor progression

Special considerations
- Follow hazardous drug guidelines for preparation and administration.
- Monitor CBC count, blood chemistries, liver function, and serum lipid levels.
- Evaluate patient regularly for chest pain and dyspnea.
- Therapy should continue even if nausea, vomiting, or diarrhea occurs.

aprepitant
Emend, Emend 3-Day

Indications and dosages
➡ Prevention of acute and delayed nausea and vomiting associated with initial and repeat courses of highly or moderately emetogenic cancer chemotherapy, including high-dose cisplatin

Adults: 125 mg P.O. 1 hour before treatment (day 1) and 80 mg once daily in morning on days 2 and 3

Special considerations
• Administer with corticosteroid and 5-HT$_3$ antagonist.
• Give with or without food.
• Long-term, continuous therapy is not recommended because drug interaction profile may change with such use.
• Administration with warfarin may significantly increase INR or prothrombin time. For patients on long-term warfarin therapy, closely monitor INR.

arsenic trioxide ⊠
Trisenox

Indications and dosages
➡ Induction of remission and consolidation of acute promyelocytic leukemia (APL) in patients who are refractory to, or have relapsed from, retinoid and anthracycline chemotherapy and whose APL is characterized by presence of t(15;17) translocation or PML/RAR-alpha gene expression
Adults: For induction, 0.15 mg/kg I.V. daily until bone marrow remission. Total induction dosage should not exceed 60 doses. For consolidation, begin 3 to 6 weeks after induction therapy ends and give 0.15 mg/kg I.V. daily for 25 doses over 5 weeks.
➡ Relapsed or refractory multiple myeloma
Adults: 0.25 mg/kg I.V. daily for 5 days for first 2 weeks of 28-day cycle
➡ Chronic myeloid leukemia in chronic, accelerated, and blast crisis
Adults: Up to 6 mg I.V. three times daily

OFF-LABEL USES (SELECTED)
➡ Myelodysplastic syndromes

Special considerations
• Follow hazardous drug guidelines for preparation and administration.
• Some patients with APL who receive drug experience symptoms similar to those of retinoic acid–acute promyelocytic leukemia or APL differentiation syndrome, which can be fatal.

⟩⟩ Potentially carcinogenic

• At first indication of APL differentiation syndrome, high-dose steroid therapy should begin immediately, irrespective of WBC count, and continue for at least 3 days until signs and symptoms have abated.

• Drug may cause complete AV block and QT interval prolongation, which can lead to potentially fatal torsade de pointes–type ventricular arrhythmia.

• Obtain baseline 12-lead ECG, creatinine level, and serum potassium, calcium, and magnesium levels before start of therapy.

• Dilute with 100 to 250 ml D_5W or normal saline injection.

• Administer I.V. over 1 to 2 hours. Infusion may last up to 4 hours if acute vasomotor reactions occur.

• Monitor electrolyte, hematologic, and coagulation profiles at least twice weekly.

• Obtain weekly ECG to check for prolonged QT interval. Initiate corrective measures for QT interval greater than 500 msec.

asparaginase ☒
Elspar

Indications and dosages

➥ Acute lymphocytic leukemia in combination with other antineoplastics

Adults: 200 international units/kg I.V. daily for 28 days, usually combined with other agents in specific regimens. Typical combination dosage is 500 mg/kg, but some regimens call for 200 mg/kg on specific days of cycle (for example, days 8, 15, 22).

Children: 6,000 international units/m² I.V. on treatment days 4, 7, 10, 13, 16, 19, 22, 25, and 28 in combination with vincristine and prednisone. Or 1,000 international units/kg daily for 10 days beginning on treatment day 22 in combination with vincristine and prednisone. When used as sole induction agent, give 200 international units/kg I.V. daily for 28 days.

Special considerations

• Follow hazardous drug guidelines for preparation and administration.

• Stop therapy permanently in patients who develop pancreatitis.

• Perform intradermal skin test before initial administration and when drug has not been given for at least 1 week.

• For I.V. use with 10,000 international unit–vials, reconstitute powder with 5 ml sterile water for injection or sodium chloride injection.
• Before infusion, dilute with normal saline solution or D$_5$W. Infuse within 8 hours.
• If administering I.M., reconstitute with 2 ml sodium chloride injection in 10,000 international unit–vial. Use within 8 hours.
• Use as sole induction agent only when combined regimen is inappropriate.
• Allergic reactions occur frequently, especially during retreatment.
• Drug may increase preexisting hepatic impairment.
• Obtain frequent serum amylase levels to detect early evidence of pancreatitis.
• Monitor blood glucose level; fatal hyperglycemia may occur.

azacitidine
Vidaza

Indications and dosages
➡ Myelodysplastic syndrome with the following subtypes: refractory anemia, refractory anemia with ringed sideroblasts (if accompanied by neutropenia or thrombocytopenia or requiring transfusions), refractory anemia with excess blasts, refractory anemia with excess blasts in transformation, and chronic myelomonocytic leukemia
Adults: 75 mg/m^2 subcutaneously daily for 7 days every 4 weeks; may increase to 100 mg/m^2 if no beneficial effect after two treatment cycles and if no toxicity other than nausea and vomiting occurs.

OFF-LABEL USES (SELECTED)
➡ Acute myeloid leukemia

Special considerations
≫ Follow hazardous drug guidelines for preparation and administration.
• Dosage adjustment is based on hematologic laboratory values, including WBC, absolute neutrophil, and platelet counts.
• If unexplained serum bicarbonate reduction to below 20 mEq/L occurs, reduce dosage by 50% for next course. If unexplained BUN or serum creatinine elevations occur, delay next cycle until values return

to normal or baseline, and reduce dosage by 50% for next treatment course.

• Obtain liver function test results and serum creatinine level before therapy begins.

• Divide doses above 4 ml equally in two syringes and inject subcutaneously in two separate sites.

• Monitor CBCs before each dosing cycle and as often as necessary between cycles.

BCG live, intravesical ☒
TheraCys, Tice BCG

Indications and dosages

➡ Prophylaxis and treatment of urinary bladder carcinoma in situ; prophylaxis of primary or recurrent stage Ta and/or T1 papillary bladder tumors after transurethral resection (TUR)

Adults: One dose (TheraCys) of 81 mg (dry weight) in 3 ml diluent provided, suspended in 50 ml preservative-free normal saline solution given intravesically once weekly for 6 weeks, then one treatment 3, 6, 12, 18, and 24 months after initial treatment; begin 7 to 14 days after TUR. Or one dose (Tice BCG) (one vial in 50 ml normal saline solution) given intravesically once weekly for 6 weeks; may repeat once; then continue monthly for 6 to 12 months; begin 7 to 14 days after TUR.

Special considerations

• Follow hazardous drug guidelines for preparation and administration.

• Drug contains live, attenuated mycobacteria.

• Before starting intravesical therapy, rule out active TB in PPD-positive patients.

• Do not give drug within 1 week of TUR.

• Postpone intravesical instillation if patient has fever or suspected infection or is receiving antimicrobials.

• Patient should not drink fluids for 4 hours before treatment, and should empty bladder before administration.

• Small bladder capacity has been associated with increased risk of severe local reactions.

☒ FDA black-box warning

- Manage bladder irritation symptomatically with phenazopyridine, propantheline, and acetaminophen.
- Watch for systemic BCG infection.

---

bevacizumab ⊠
Avastin

Indications and dosages

➥ Metastatic colon or rectal carcinoma (in combination with I.V. 5-fluorouracil-based chemotherapy)

Adults: 5 mg/kg by I.V. infusion once every 14 days until disease progression occurs. Do not start therapy for at least 28 days after major surgery and until surgical incision is fully healed.

OFF-LABEL USES (SELECTED)

➥ Breast cancer
➥ Non-small-cell lung cancer, first-line treatment in combination with paclitaxel and carboplatin for advanced or metastatic non-squamous-cell disease

Special considerations

- Discontinue drug permanently in patients with hypertensive crisis and temporarily in those with severe hypertension.
- Regularly monitor patients with moderate to severe proteinuria.
- GI perforation and wound dehiscence, complicated by intra-abdominal abscesses, have occurred.
- Serious and fatal hemoptysis has occurred in patients with non-small-cell lung cancer treated with bevacizumab.
- Do not administer or mix infusions with dextrose solutions.
- Do not give as I.V. push or bolus. Deliver initial dose over 90 minutes as I.V. infusion. If first infusion is well tolerated, may administer second infusion over 60 minutes; if well tolerated, may administer all subsequent infusions over 30 minutes.
- Drug may impair wound healing.
- Before each dose, monitor urine protein with serial urinalyses for development or worsening of proteinuria.
- Monitor blood pressure throughout therapy.

▶▶ Potentially carcinogenic

bexarotene ⊠
Targretin

Indications and dosages

➡ Cutaneous manifestations of cutaneous T-cell lymphoma in patients refractory to at least one previous systemic therapy

Adults: 300 mg/m² P.O.daily.

➡ Treatment of cutaneous lesions in patients with cutaneous T-cell lymphoma (stage IA and IB) who have refractory or persistent disease after other therapies or who have not tolerated other therapies

Adults: Gel applied topically once every other day for first week, increased at weekly intervals up to four times daily, according to individual lesion tolerance

Special considerations

• Follow hazardous drug guidelines for preparation and administration.

• Oral dosage may be adjusted to 200 mg/m² daily and then 100 mg/m² daily if necessitated by toxicity or increased liver function test values.

• If no tumor response occurs after 8 weeks of treatment, dosage may be increased to 400 mg/m² daily with careful monitoring.

• If severe local irritation occurs with topical application, dosage can be reduced or drug temporarily discontinued.

• Capsules are a member of retinoid class associated with birth defects and must not be given to pregnant women.

• Obtain baseline liver function test results before administering drug.

• Measure blood lipid levels before administering.

• Apply sufficient gel to cover lesion generously. Allow gel to dry before covering with clothing.

• Obtain baseline WBC count with differential and periodically during treatment.

• Carefully monitor liver function tests after 1, 2, and 4 weeks of treatment.

• Consider thyroid hormone supplements for patients with laboratory evidence of hypothyroidism.

• Monitor for and treat major lipid abnormalities that occur during long-term therapy.

bicalutamide
Casodex

Indications and dosages
➡ Stage D$_2$ metastatic carcinoma of prostate (in combination with luteinizing hormone–releasing hormone [LH-RH] analogue)
Adults: One 50-mg tablet P.O. once daily

Special considerations
• Follow hazardous drug guidelines for preparation and administration.
• Measure serum transaminase levels before, during, and after treatment.
• Drug is given with LH-RH analogue, starting at same time.
• Evaluate serum prostate specific antigen regularly.
• If patient develops hepatic dysfunction, measure serum transaminase levels immediately. If jaundice occurs or ALT level rises above 2 × ULN, discontinue drug immediately.
• Drug can displace coumarin anticoagulants such as warfarin from protein-binding sites.

bleomycin sulfate ⊠
Blenoxane

Indications and dosages
➡ Squamous-cell carcinoma, non-Hodgkin's lymphoma
Adults and adolescents: 0.25 to 0.5 unit/kg (10 to 20 units/m^2) I.V., I.M., or subcutaneously weekly or twice weekly
➡ Testicular carcinoma
Adults: 0.25 to 0.5 unit/kg (10 to 20 units/m^2) I.V., I.M., or subcutaneously weekly or twice weekly. In BEP regimen, bleomycin 30 units I.V. on days 2, 9, and 16, with etoposide 100 mg/m^2 on days 1 to 5, and cisplatin 20 mg/m^2 on days 1 to 5; repeated every 21 days
➡ Hodgkin's disease
Adults and adolescents: 0.25 to 0.5 unit/kg (10 to 20 units/m^2) I.V., I.M., or subcutaneously weekly or twice weekly; then, after 50% response, maintenance dosage of 1 unit daily or 5 units weekly I.V. or I.M. In ABVD regimen, doxorubicin 25 mg/m^2, bleomycin 10 units/m^2,

⯈⯈ Potentially carcinogenic

vinblastine 6 mg/m², and dacarbazine 375 mg/m² I.V. on days 1 and 15; repeated every 28 days.

➥ Malignant pleural effusion

Adults and adolescents: 60 units in 50 to 100 ml normal saline solution given as a single-dose bolus intrapleural injection

Off-label uses (selected)

➥ Cutaneous malignancies (basal-cell carcinoma, squamous-cell carcinoma, advanced metastatic melanoma, Kaposi's sarcoma)

Special considerations

⏩ Follow hazardous drug guidelines for preparation and administration.

• If no acute reaction occurs, follow regular dosage schedule.

• Some practitioners limit total lifetime dose to 300 to 400 units because of risk of pulmonary toxicity.

• Patients with moderate renal failure (glomerular filtration rate [GFR] of 10 to 50 ml/minute) should receive 75% of usual dose at normal dosage interval; patients with severe renal failure (GFR below 10 ml/minute) should receive 50% of usual dose at normal dosage interval.

• Pulmonary fibrosis is most severe toxicity.

• Severe idiosyncratic reaction—consisting of hypotension, mental confusion, fever, chills, and wheezing—may occur after first or second dose. A test dose is recommended for high-risk patients.

• Premedicate with acetaminophen, corticosteroids, and diphenhydramine to prevent fever and decrease risk of anaphylaxis.

• Reconstitute 15-unit vial with 1 to 5 ml sterile water for injection, normal saline solution for injection, or sterile bacteriostatic water for injection. Reconstitute 30-unit vial with 2 to 10 ml of above diluents.

• For I.V. injection, dissolve contents of 15- or 30-unit vial in 5 ml or 10 ml, respectively, of normal saline solution for injection. Administer slowly over 10 minutes.

• For intermittent infusion, dilute further and infuse over 15 minutes or longer.

• For intrapleural use, dissolve 60 units in 50 to 100 ml normal saline injection, and administer through thoracostomy tube after drainage of excess pleural fluid and confirmation of complete lung expansion.

• Clamp thoracostomy tube after instillation. Move patient from supine to left and right lateral positions several times over next 4 hours. Remove clamp and reestablish suction. Length of time chest tube remains in place after sclerosis depends on clinical situation.

• Evaluate respiratory status regularly.

• Monitor renal function, chest X-ray, and pulmonary status throughout therapy.

---

bortezomib
Velcade

Indications and dosages

➡ Multiple myeloma in patients who have received at least one previous therapy

Adults: Standard schedule is 1.3 mg/m^2 as bolus I.V. injection over 3 to 5 seconds twice weekly for 2 weeks (days 1, 4, 8, and 11), followed by 10-day rest period (days 12 to 21); repeated every 21 days as tolerated. For therapy of more than 8 weeks, give on standard schedule or maintenance schedule of once weekly for 4 weeks (days 1, 8, 15, and 22) followed by 13-day rest period (days 23 to 35). Allow at least 72 hours between consecutive doses.

OFF-LABEL USES (SELECTED)

➡ Relapsed, refractory non-Hodgkin's lymphoma (primarily mantle-cell lymphoma)

Special considerations

• Discontinue temporarily if patient experiences Grade 4 thrombocytopenia.

• Withhold drug at onset of Grade 3 nonhematologic or Grade 4 hematologic toxicities, excluding neuropathy.

• Administer fluid and electrolyte replacement to prevent dehydration.

• Reconstitute each vial with 3.5 ml normal saline injection for a concentration of 1 mg/ml.

• Administer by I.V. bolus over 3 to 5 seconds.

• Allow 72 hours between consecutive doses.

• Monitor CBCs (including platelet counts) frequently.

• Drug causes peripheral neuropathy that is predominantly sensory but may be mixed sensorimotor.

▶▶ Potentially carcinogenic

busulfan ⊠
Busulfex, Myleran

Indications and dosages
➡ Conditioning regimen before allogeneic hematopoietic progenitor cell transplantation for chronic myelogenous leukemia (in combination with cyclophosphamide)

Adults: 0.8 mg/kg of ideal body weight (IBW) or actual weight (whichever is lower) I.V. every 6 hours for 4 days (total of 16 doses) as 2-hour infusion through central venous catheter. Cyclophosphamide 60 mg/kg is given on each of 2 days as 1-hour I.V. infusion, starting 3 days before bone marrow transplant day and no sooner than 6 hours after 16th busulfan dose.

➡ Palliative treatment of chronic myelogenous (myeloid, myelocytic, or granulocytic) leukemia

Adults and children: For remission induction, approximately 60 mcg/kg or 1.8 mg/m^2 (for adults, usually 4 to 8 mg) P.O.; reserve dosages above 4 mg daily for patients with most compelling symptoms. With remission of less than 3 months, maintenance therapy of 1 to 3 mg P.O. daily may be advisable to control hematologic status and prevent rapid relapse.

OFF-LABEL USES (SELECTED)

➡ Conditioning regimen for children before allogeneic hematopoietic progenitor-cell transplantation for various malignant hematologic diseases (in combination with cyclophosphamide)

Special considerations
》》 Follow hazardous drug guidelines for preparation and administration.

• For obese or severely obese patients, administer drug based on adjusted IBW.

• With remission of less than 3 months, maintenance dosage of 1 to 3 mg daily may control hematologic status and prevent rapid relapse.

• Drug effects may be delayed.

• WBC count may increase, which does not indicate drug resistance or warrant dosage increase.

⊠ FDA black-box warning

- Because WBC count may decrease for more than 1 month after therapy ends, drug must be discontinued before total WBC count falls to normal range.
- Always premedicate with phenytoin.
- Give antiemetics before initial dose and continue throughout treatment.
- Dilute solution with either normal saline solution for injection or D_5W injection to a diluent:drug ratio of 10:1.
- Give I.V. through central venous catheter as 2-hour infusion.
- Total WBC count declines exponentially with constant busulfan dose.
- Severe granulocytopenia, thrombocytopenia, anemia, or combination may occur. Monitor CBCs and quantitative platelet counts frequently.
- Drug may cause cellular dysplasia in lungs and other organs.

capecitabine ⊠
Xeloda

Indications and dosages

➡ Metastatic colorectal carcinoma when treatment with a fluoropyrimidine such as capecitabine alone is preferred

Adults: 1,250 mg/m² P.O. twice daily (morning and evening; 2,500 mg/m² total daily dose) for 2 weeks followed by 1-week rest, given as 3-week cycles

➡ Metastatic breast cancer resistant to both paclitaxel and anthracycline-containing chemotherapy regimen or resistant to paclitaxel and when further anthracycline therapy is not indicated (monotherapy) or after failure of previous anthracycline-containing chemotherapy (combination therapy with docetaxel)

Adults: As single agent, 1,250 mg/m² P.O. twice daily (morning and evening) for 2 weeks followed by 1-week rest, given as 3-week cycles. Alternatively, 1,250 mg/m² P.O. twice daily for 2 weeks followed by 1-week rest, in combination with docetaxel 75 mg/m² as 1-hour I.V. infusion every 3 weeks

Off-label uses (selected)

➡ Colorectal cancer
➡ Renal cell carcinoma

Special considerations
- Follow hazardous drug guidelines for preparation and administration.
- For patients with moderate renal impairment, reduce dosage to 75% of starting dose.
- If Grade 2 or 3 hand-and-foot syndrome occurs, interrupt therapy until event resolves or decreases to Grade 1.
- If drug-related Grade 2 to 4 elevations in bilirubin occur, interrupt therapy until hyperbilirubinemia resolves or decreases to Grade 1.
- Altered coagulation parameters, bleeding, and death have occurred in patients taking drug concomitantly with coumarin-derivative anticoagulants.
- Premedicate according to product label before giving to patients receiving capecitabine-docetaxel combination.
- Give with water within 30 minutes after meals.

carboplatin ⊠
Paraplatin

Indications and dosages
➥ Advanced ovarian cancer (combined with cyclophosphamide)
Adults: 300 mg/m^2 I.V. (with 600 mg/m^2 cyclophosphamide) I.V. on day 1 every 4 weeks for six cycles
➥ Ovarian cancer recurring after chemotherapy
Adults: 360 mg/m^2 I.V. on day 1 every 4 weeks

Off-label uses (selected)
➥ Bladder cancer
➥ Non-small-cell lung cancer
➥ Small-cell lung cancer

Special considerations
- Follow hazardous drug guidelines for preparation and administration.
- Adjust dosage according to platelet and neutrophil counts.
- For creatinine clearance of 41 to 59 ml/minute, adjust day-1 dosage to 250 mg/m^2. For creatinine clearance of 16 to 40 ml/minute, adjust day-1 dosage to 200 mg/m^2.
- Use formula dosing based on estimates of glomerular filtration rate in elderly patients.

⊠ FDA black-box warning

• Emesis may be more severe in patients who previously received emetogenic therapy.

• Dilute each 10 mg with 1 ml sterile water for injection, D_5W, or normal saline solution. Further dilute with normal saline solution or D_5W to 1 to 4 mg/ml.

• Infuse for 15 minutes or longer.

• Bone marrow depression is a dose-dependent and dose-limiting toxicity. Monitor peripheral blood counts during therapy

• Some patients may need transfusions during treatment.

• Vision loss has been reported with doses higher than those recommended in package insert. Significant hearing loss has occurred in children who received higher-than-recommended doses combined with other ototoxic agents.

• High doses have caused severe liver function abnormalities.

• Creatinine clearance is most sensitive measure of renal function, and is most useful test for correlating drug clearance with bone marrow depression.

carmustine (BCNU) ⊠
BiCNU, Gliadel

Indications and dosages

➡ Palliative therapy (as single agent or in combination) for glioblastoma, brainstem glioma, medulloblastoma, astrocytoma, ependymoma, metastatic brain tumors, and multiple myeloma (in combination with prednisone); secondary palliative therapy in Hodgkin's disease and non-Hodgkin's lymphoma (in combination with other approved drugs) in patients who relapse during or fail to respond to primary therapy
Adults: 150 to 200 mg/m² I.V. infusion over 1 to 2 hours every 6 weeks (as single agent in previously untreated patients) as single dose or divided into daily injections, such as 75 to 100 mg/m² on 2 successive days
➡ Newly diagnosed high-grade malignant glioma as adjunct to surgery and radiation, or recurrent glioblastoma multiforme as adjunct to surgery
Adults: 61.6 mg (eight wafers) by implantation into resection cavity, if size and shape allow

---

⟫ Potentially carcinogenic

➥ Disseminated malignant melanoma

Special considerations

>> Follow hazardous drug guidelines for preparation and administration.

• Adjust dosage when drug is combined with other myelosuppressants and in patients with depleted bone marrow reserve.

• Do not give repeat carmustine course until circulating blood elements have returned to acceptable levels (platelets above 100,000/mm³ and WBCs above 4,000/mm³).

• Bone marrow toxicity is cumulative, and adjustment must be considered on basis of nadir blood counts with previous dose.

• Patients receiving more than 1,400 mg/m² cumulative dose are at significantly higher risk for pulmonary toxicity.

• Administer antiemetic 30 to 60 minutes before drug.

• Dissolve drug with 3 ml supplied sterile diluent (dehydrated alcohol injection). Add 27 ml sterile water for injection.

• May be diluted further with 5% dextrose injection.

• Do not administer over less than 1 to 2 hours, to avoid intense pain and burning at injection site (although true thrombosis is rare).

• Pouches containing wafers should remain unopened until implantation. Up to eight implants may be placed to cover as much of resection cavity as possible. Slight overlapping is acceptable. Wafers broken in half may be used, but those broken into more than two pieces should be discarded in biohazard container. Oxidized regenerated cellulose (Surgicel) may cover wafers to secure them against cavity surface. After placement, irrigate resection cavity and close dura in watertight fashion.

• Monitor platelet, WBC, and neutrophil counts weekly for acceptable levels.

• Do not give repeat course before 6 weeks because hematologic toxicity is delayed and cumulative.

• Monitor liver and kidney function tests periodically.

• CT scans and MRI of head may show enhancement in brain tissue surrounding resection cavity after implantation. This may represent edema and inflammation caused by implant or tumor progression.

cetuximab ⊠
Erbitux

Indications and dosages
➡ Epidermal growth factor receptor (EGFR)–expressing, metastatic colorectal cancer in patients refractory to irinotecan-based chemotherapy (in combination with irinotecan); EGFR-expressing, metastatic colorectal cancer in patients intolerant of irinotecan-based chemotherapy (single agent)

Adults: 400 mg/m^2 as initial loading dose by I.V. infusion over 2 hours (maximum infusion rate is 5 ml/minute), and weekly maintenance dose of 250 mg/m^2 infused over 1 hour (maximum infusion rate is 5 ml/minute)

Off-label uses (selected)
➡ Relapsed or refractory head and neck cancer
➡ Breast cancer
➡ Tumors overexpressing EGFR

Special considerations
• If patient experiences mild or moderate (Grade 1 or 2) infusion reaction, permanently reduce infusion rate by 50%.
• For severe acneiform rash, delay infusion 1 to 2 weeks. If condition improves, continue therapy at reduced dosage. If no improvement occurs, discontinue therapy.
• Premedicate with a histamine$_1$ antagonist.
• Do not reconstitute.
• Administer initial dose over 2 hours at rate of 5 ml/minute; give subsequent weekly doses over 1 hour. Maximum infusion rate is 5 ml/minute.
• Observe patient for 1 hour after infusion. Severe, potentially fatal infusion reactions have occurred.
• Watch for interstitial lung disease.
• Incidence and severity of cutaneous reactions with combined-modality therapy appear to be additive.

⨠ Potentially carcinogenic

chlorambucil ☒
Leukeran

Indications and dosages
➥ Chronic lymphocytic leukemia (CLL); malignant lymphomas, including lymphosarcoma, giant follicular lymphoma, and Hodgkin's disease

Adults: 0.1 to 0.2 mg/kg P.O. daily for 3 to 6 weeks to response or bone marrow depression

OFF-LABEL USES (SELECTED)

➥ Combination therapy for Hodgkin's disease

Special considerations
⟫ Follow hazardous drug guidelines for preparation and administration.

• Carefully adjust dosage to patient response; reduce as soon as WBC count falls abruptly. Patients with Hodgkin's disease usually require 0.2 mg/kg daily; patients with other lymphomas or CLL usually require 0.1 mg/kg daily.

• Drug should not be given at full dosages before 4 weeks after full course of radiation therapy or chemotherapy because of possible bone marrow vulnerability to damage.

• If bone marrow infiltration is confirmed or bone marrow is hypoplastic, daily dosage should not exceed 0.1 mg/kg.

• Decrease dosage if WBC or platelet count falls below normal.

• Entire daily dose may be given at once.

• Drug may be given at bedtime and with antiemetic to limit GI effects.

• Seizures, infertility, leukemia, and secondary malignancies have occurred.

• Monitor patient carefully to avoid life-threatening bone marrow damage. Test blood weekly for hemoglobin, total and differential WBC counts, and quantitative platelet counts.

• Slowly progressive lymphopenia develops during treatment. Lymphocyte count usually returns to normal rapidly when therapy ends.

• Neutropenia usually develops after third week of treatment and may last up to 10 days after last dose.

cisplatin ☒
Platinol-AQ

Indications and dosages
➡ Metastatic testicular cancer (in combination with other approved chemotherapeutic agents)
Adults: 20 mg/m^2 I.V. daily for 5 days
➡ Metastatic ovarian cancer (in combination with cyclophosphamide)
Adults: 75 to 100 mg/m^2 I.V. once every 4 weeks
➡ Metastatic ovarian cancer refractory to standard chemotherapy in patients who have not previously received cisplatin (monotherapy)
Adults: 100 mg/m^2 I.V. once every 4 weeks
➡ Advanced bladder cancer (monotherapy)
Adults: 50 to 70 mg/m^2 I.V. once every 3 to 4 weeks depending on extent of previous exposure to radiation or chemotherapy. For heavily pretreated patients, give 50 mg/m^2 repeated every 4 weeks.

OFF-LABEL USES (SELECTED)

➡ Soft-tissue sarcoma, mesothelioma, melanoma, osteosarcoma of unknown primary origin, salvage treatment of lymphomas, bone marrow transplant conditioning regimens

Special considerations
》 Follow hazardous drug guidelines for preparation and administration.
• Do not give initial or repeat doses unless serum creatinine level is below 1.5 mg/100 ml or BUN level is below 25 mg/100 ml, platelet count is at least 100,000/mm^3, and WBC count is at least 4,000/mm^3.
• Before giving dose, hydrate patient with 1 to 2 L fluid infused over 8 to 12 hours.
• Platinol AQ is prediluted to 1 mg/ml. Initially, dilute each 50-mg vial with 50 ml sterile water for injection to yield 1 mg/ml. Immediately before use, further dilute each half of single dose in 1 L 5% dextrose in one-quarter or one-half normal saline solution, or normal saline solution containing 12.5 to 25 g mannitol. Do not use D$_5$W.
• Infuse each 1 L of solution over 3 to 4 hours.
• Anaphylactoid-like reactions to cisplatin have occurred within minutes of administration in patients with previous exposure.

》 Potentially carcinogenic

• Severe neuropathies have occurred with dosages and dosing frequencies greater than recommended.

• Monitor kidney function tests frequently and peripheral blood counts weekly. Periodically monitor liver function tests, and regularly perform neurologic examinations.

• Perform audiometric testing before initiating therapy and before each subsequent dose because drug's ototoxicity is cumulative.

cladribine ⊠
Cladribine Novaplus, Leustatin

Indications and dosages

➥ Active hairy cell leukemia
Adults: 0.09 mg/kg continuous I.V. infusion over 24 hours as single course for 7 consecutive days

OFF-LABEL USES (SELECTED)

➥ Active hairy cell leukemia
➥ Cutaneous T-cell lymphoma, chronic lymphocytic leukemia, non-Hodgkin's lymphoma
➥ Acute myeloid leukemia

Special considerations

• Follow hazardous drug guidelines for preparation and administration.
• Consider delaying or discontinuing therapy if neurotoxicity or renal toxicity occurs.
• For patients taking blood dyscrasia–causing drugs, base dosage adjustment on hematologic parameters.
• Dosage reduction may be needed when two or more bone marrow depressants (including radiation) are used concurrently or consecutively with cladribine.
• Drug is approved for I.V. infusion only.
• Dilute with designated diluent.
• Solution is incompatible with D_5W.
• To prepare single daily dose, add calculated dose to infusion bag containing 500 ml normal saline for injection.
• Don't mix solution with other I.V. drugs or additives or infuse simultaneously through common I.V. line.

• Benzyl alcohol (constituent of recommended diluent for 7-day infusion) has been linked to fatal "gasping syndrome" in premature infants.
• To prepare 7-day ambulatory continuous I.V. infusion, use bacteriostatic normal saline solution and sterile 0.22-micron filter. Admixtures for 7-day infusion are stable for at least 7 days.
• Closely monitor patient for hematologic and nonhematologic toxicity.
• Monitor renal and hepatic function.
• Febrile episodes are common and can occur anytime but typically appear 3 to 4 days into therapy (possibly from cytokine release).

clofarabine
Clolar

Indications and dosages
➥ Relapsed or refractory acute lymphoblastic leukemia after at least two previous regimens
Children ages 1 to adults age 21: 52 mg/m^2 by I.V. infusion over 2 hours daily for 5 consecutive days every 2 to 6 weeks, depending on toxicity and response

OFF-LABEL USES (SELECTED)

➥ Relapsed or refractory acute myeloid leukemia in children
➥ Relapsed or refractory acute leukemias

Special considerations
• Repeat treatment cycles after recovery or return to baseline organ function, about every 2 to 6 weeks. Base dosage on patient's body surface area, calculated using height and weight before start of each cycle.
• Discontinue drug immediately if patient has significant signs or symptoms (such as hypotension) of systemic inflammatory response syndrome (SIRS) or capillary leak syndrome (CLS).
• If creatinine or bilirubin levels rise significantly, discontinue drug.
• Evaluate hepatic and renal function before and during treatment. Closely monitor respiratory status and blood pressure during infusion.
• Filter through sterile 0.22-micron syringe filter; then further dilute with D$_5$W or normal saline for injection before I.V. infusion.
• Give continuous I.V. fluids throughout 5 days of treatment to reduce effects of tumor lysis and other adverse events.

>> Potentially carcinogenic

• Monitor patient for tumor lysis syndrome or cytokine release that could develop into SIRS, CLS, or organ dysfunction.

• Monitor hematologic status and renal and hepatic function closely.

• ALT and AST elevations are transient; they typically occur within 1 week of administration and last less than 2 weeks.

---

cyclophosphamide
Cytoxan, Cytoxan Lyophilized, Neosar

Indications and dosages

➥ Malignant lymphomas (Stages III and IV of Ann Arbor system), Hodgkin's disease, lymphocytic lymphoma (nodular or diffuse), mixed-cell type lymphoma, histiocytic lymphoma, Burkitt's lymphoma, multiple myeloma, chronic lymphocytic leukemia, chronic granulocytic leukemia, acute myelogenous and monocytic leukemia, acute lymphoblastic (stem cell) leukemia in children, mycosis fungoides (advanced), neuroblastoma (disseminated), ovarian adenocarcinoma, retinoblastoma, carcinoma of breast

Adults and children: 40 to 50 mg/kg I.V. in divided doses over 2 to 5 days; or 10 to 15 mg/kg I.V. every 7 to 10 days; or 3 to 5 mg/kg I.V. twice weekly; or 1 to 5 mg/kg P.O. daily for initial and maintenance dosing

OFF-LABEL USES (SELECTED)

➥ Breast, ovarian, cervical, bladder, head and neck, prostrate, and lung cancer (usually small-cell); Ewing's sarcoma

Special considerations

▶▶ Follow hazardous drug guidelines for preparation and administration.

• Adjust dosage based on antitumor activity or leukopenia.

• After adrenalectomy, dosages of both replacement steroids and cyclophosphamide may need adjustment.

• For patients taking blood dyscrasia–causing drugs, dosage may need adjustment based on hematologic parameters.

• Dosage reduction may be required for patients receiving two or more bone marrow depressants concurrently or consecutively.

• Consider dosage adjustment in patients with renal or hepatic insufficiency.

• Serious and sometimes fatal infections may develop in severely immunosuppressed patients.
• Dilute each 100 mg with 5 ml sterile water for injection. May further dilute with 100 to 250 ml D_5W, normal saline solution, 5% dextrose in normal saline solution, or lactated Ringer's solution.
• Drug may be given by I.V. push (each 100 mg given over 1 minute).
• Intermittent infusion is recommended for doses above 500 mg. Dilute with 100 to 250 ml D_5W, normal saline solution, 5% dextrose in normal saline solution, or lactated Ringer's solution; give over 20 to 60 minutes.
• Drug has caused secondary cancers (most commonly urinary bladder, myeloproliferative, or lymphoproliferative).
• Hemorrhagic cystitis may occur, which may be severe and even fatal (though rarely).

cytarabine ⊠
Cytosar-U

cytarabine liposome ⊠
DepoCyt

Indications and dosages
➥ Remission induction in acute nonlymphocytic leukemia (used in combination)
Adults and children: 100 mg/m² daily (conventional form) by continuous I.V. infusion (days 1 to 7) or 100 mg/m² (conventional form) I.V. every 12 hours (days 1 to 7)
➥ Postremission therapy in acute nonlymphocytic leukemia (used in combination)
Adults and children: 1 to 3 g/m² (conventional form) I.V. infusion over 1 to 3 hours every 12 hours for 3 to 6 days. Most common regimen is 3 g/m² daily (conventional form) infused over 3 hours every 12 hours on days 1, 3, and 5 for six doses in patients younger than age 60.
➥ Acute lymphocytic leukemia
Adults and children: For multidose strategies, see specific regimens. High-dose cytarabine (conventional form) is given as 1 to 3 g/m² I.V. piggyback over 1 to 3 hours for 2 to 4 doses. For induction phase, 75 to 150 mg/m² (conventional form) I.V. daily on designated days.

⟫⟫ Potentially carcinogenic

➥ Blast phase of chronic myelocytic leukemia

Adults and children: Treat as for acute leukemia. See specific regimen.

➥ Prophylaxis and treatment of meningeal leukemia

Adults: 5 to 75 mg/m^2 intrathecally once daily for 4 days or once every 4 days until cerebrospinal fluid (CSF) findings are normal, followed by one additional treatment (conventional form). Alternative treatment schedule is twice weekly (conventional form) until CSF clears, then weekly for 4 weeks. However, multiple strategies exist.

➥ Lymphomatous meningitis

Adults: For induction therapy, 50 mg (liposomal form) intrathecally (intraventricular or lumbar puncture) every 14 days for two doses (weeks 1 and 3); for consolidation therapy, 50 mg (liposomal form) intrathecally (intraventricular or lumbar puncture) every 14 days for three doses (weeks 5, 7, and 9), followed by one additional dose at week 13. For maintenance, 50 mg (liposomal form) intrathecally (intraventricular or lumbar puncture) every 28 days for four doses (weeks 17, 21, 25, and 29). Give dexamethasone 4 mg P.O. or I.V. twice daily for 5 days, starting on day of liposome injection, with each treatment.

OFF-LABEL USES (SELECTED)

➥ Hodgkin's and non-Hodgkin's lymphoma

Special considerations

• Follow hazardous drug guidelines for preparation and administration.
• If drug-induced neurotoxicity develops, reduce dosage to 25 mg. If neurotoxicity persists, discontinue drug.
• Dosage reduction may be required when two or more bone marrow depressants (including radiation) are used concurrently or consecutively.
• Consider suspending drug or modifying therapy if drug-induced bone marrow depression results in platelet count below 50,000/mm^3 or polymorphonuclear granulocyte count below 1,000/mm^3.
• Monitor patient closely. Frequent platelet and WBC counts and bone marrow examinations are mandatory.
• Periodically check liver and kidney function test results.
• Perform neurologic evaluations and cerebellar assessment in patients receiving high doses.

Cytarabine

• Give dexamethasone eyedrops before high-dose cytarabine, and continue for at least 24 hours after administration to prevent conjunctivitis.

⊠ FDA black-box warning

- High-dose cytarabine is highly emetogenic; use aggressive antiemetic therapy.
- Reconstitute each 100 mg with 5 ml bacteriostatic water for injection for I.V. infusion.
- For intrathecal administration, reconstitute with preservative-free normal saline solution for injection; use immediately.
- For I.V. infusion, may further dilute with normal saline solution or D_5W and give over 30 minutes to 24 hours.

Cytarabine liposome
- Administer dexamethasone 4 mg twice daily P.O. or I.V. for 5 days, starting on day of liposome injection.
- Administer by intrathecal route only. Further dilution is not recommended.
- Withdraw from vial immediately before administration and use within 4 hours.
- Administer directly into CSF through intraventricular reservoir or by direct injection into lumbar sac. Inject slowly over 1 to 5 minutes. After administration by lumbar puncture, instruct patient to lie flat for 1 hour.

dacarbazine (DTIC) ⊠
DTIC-Dome

Indications and dosages
➡ Metastatic malignant melanoma
Adults: 2 to 4.5 mg/kg I.V. daily for 10 days, repeated at 4-week intervals; or 250 mg/m² I.V. daily for 5 days, repeated every 3 weeks. Or, in CVD regimen (cisplatin, vinblastine, and dacarbazine), 800 mg/m² I.V. on day 1, repeated every 21 days.
➡ Hodgkin's lymphoma
Adults: 150 mg/m² I.V. for 5 days in combination with other effective drugs, repeated every 4 weeks. Or 375 mg/m² I.V. on day 1 in combination with other effective drugs every 15 days (ABVD regimen).

OFF-LABEL USES (SELECTED)

➡ Soft-tissue sarcoma
➡ Islet-cell carcinoma and carcinoid tumors
➡ Malignant pheochromocytoma

⟫ Potentially carcinogenic

Special considerations

▷▷ Follow hazardous drug guidelines for preparation and administration.

• Reduce dosage in patients with impaired renal and hepatic function.

• Give prophylactic antiemetics. Prophylactic antibiotics may be indicated for febrile neutropenic patient.

• Reconstitute with sterile water for injection to yield 10 mg/ml.

• Reconstituted solution may be diluted further with 50 to 250 ml D_5W or normal saline solution, and given as I.V. infusion.

• Infuse total dose over 30 to 60 minutes.

• Possibility of bone marrow depression necessitates careful WBC, RBC, and platelet monitoring.

---

dactinomycin (ACT, actinomycin D) ⊠
Cosmegen

Indications and dosages

➡ Wilms' tumor, childhood rhabdomyosarcoma, Ewing's sarcoma (combination therapy)
Children: 15 mcg/kg I.V. daily for 5 days given in various combinations and schedules with other chemotherapeutic agents (not to exceed 0.5 mg/day)

➡ Metastatic nonseminomatous testicular cancer
Adults: 1,000 mcg/m^2 I.V. on day 1 as part of combination regimen with cyclophosphamide, bleomycin, vinblastine, and cisplatin

➡ Gestational trophoblastic neoplasia (monotherapy or combination therapy)
Adults: 12 mcg/kg I.V. daily for 5 days as single agent. Or 500 mcg I.V. on days 1 and 2 as part of combination regimen with etoposide, methotrexate, folinic acid, vincristine, cyclophosphamide, and cisplatin.

➡ Locally recurrent or locoregional solid cancers
Adults: 50 mcg (0.05 mg)/kg I.V. for lower extremity or pelvis; 35 mcg (0.035 mg)/kg I.V. for upper extremity

➡ Osteosarcoma
Adults: 0.6 mg/m^2 I.V. for 2 days on weeks 2, 13, 26, 39, and 42 after surgery. Used in combination with high-dose methotrexate (12 g/m^2).

Special considerations

- Follow hazardous drug guidelines for preparation and administration.
- For patients taking blood dyscrasia–causing drugs, base dosage adjustment on hematologic parameters.
- Reduce dosage in patients with hyperbilirubinemia.
- Antiemetics are given before therapy begins.
- Do not give I.M. or subcutaneously.
- Dilute each 0.5-mg vial with preservative-free sterile water for injection to yield 0.5 mg/ml. May further dilute with 50 ml D_5W or normal saline solution.
- Give single I.V. dose by injection over 2 to 3 minutes. Give single I.V. dose by infusion over 20 to 30 minutes.
- Frequently evaluate renal, hepatic, and bone marrow function.
- Incidence of second primary tumors may increase after therapy.
- Administer extremely cautiously within 2 months of radiation therapy for right-sided Wilms' tumor.

darbepoetin alfa
Aranesp

Indications and dosages

➡ Anemia in patients with nonmyeloid malignancies when anemia results from concomitant chemotherapy
Adults: 2.25 mcg/kg subcutaneously given as weekly injection

OFF-LABEL USES (SELECTED)

➡ Anemia associated with chemotherapy

Special considerations

- Adjust dosage to achieve and maintain target hemoglobin no higher than 12 g/dl.
- For patients who respond to drug with rapid increase in hemoglobin, reduce dosage.
- Closely monitor and control blood pressure.
- Do not increase dosage more frequently than once a month.
- Evaluate iron status before and during treatment.
- Darbepoetin alfa and other erythropoietic therapies may increase risk of cardiovascular events.

⟫ Potentially carcinogenic

- Closely monitor renal function and fluid and electrolyte balance.
- Drug increases RBCs and decreases plasma volume.

---

daunorubicin citrate liposome ⊠
DaunoXome

Indications and dosages
➥ Advanced HIV-associated Kaposi's sarcoma
Adults: 40 mg/m^2 I.V. over 60 minutes, with doses repeated every 2 weeks; total dose not to exceed 400 mg/m^2

Off-label uses (selected)

➥ Acute leukemias
➥ Multiple myeloma
➥ Metastatic colon cancer, adjunct in lymphoma

Special considerations
▷▷ Follow hazardous drug guidelines for preparation and administration.
- Determine blood counts before each dose. Withhold drug if absolute granulocyte count is less than 750 cells/mm^3.
- For patients with serum bilirubin level of 1.2 to 3 mg/dl, reduce usual dosage by 25%; if serum bilirubin or creatinine level exceeds 3 mg/dl, reduce usual dosage by 50%.
- Dosage reduction may be required when two or more bone marrow depressants (including radiation) are used concurrently or consecutively with this drug.
- Triad of back pain, flushing, and chest tightness has occurred and usually arises during first 5 minutes of infusion, subsides with interruption of infusion, and does not recur if infusion resumes at slower rate.
- Dilute single dose with equal amount of D$_5$W to yield 1 mg/ml.
- Transfer to infusion bag containing equal volume of D$_5$W and infuse over 60 minutes.
- Careful hematologic monitoring is required for bone marrow depression; patient must be observed carefully for evidence of intercurrent or opportunistic infections.
- Carefully evaluate cardiac function.

⊠ FDA black-box warning

daunorubicin hydrochloride ⊠
Cerubidine

Indications and dosages
➥ Acute nonlymphocytic leukemia
Adults: 45 mg/m² I.V. daily on days 1, 2, and 3 of first course and days 1 and 2 of subsequent courses, and cytosine arabinoside 100 mg/m² I.V. infusion daily for 7 days for first course and for 5 days for subsequent courses, if required
➥ Acute lymphocytic leukemia
Adults: 45 mg/m² I.V. daily on days 1, 2, and 3 and vincristine 2 mg I.V. on days 1, 8, and 15, and prednisone 40 mg/m² P.O. daily on days 1 to 22, then tapered between days 22 and 29; L-asparaginase 500 international units/kg daily for 10 days on days 22 to 32
Children older than age 2: 25 mg/m² I.V. on day 1 every week, vincristine 1.5 mg/m² I.V. on day 1 every week, prednisone 40 mg/m² P.O. daily. (Multiple dosing strategies exist; see specific regimens.)

OFF-LABEL USES (SELECTED)

➥ Chronic myelogenous leukemia in blastic phase

Special considerations
≫ Follow hazardous drug guidelines for preparation and administration.
• Reduce dosage in patients with hepatic or renal impairment.
• For patients age 60 and older, reduce dosage to 30 mg/m² daily and use same regimen as for patients younger than age 60.
• For children younger than age 2 or less than 0.5 m² body surface area (BSA), base dosage on weight (1 mg/kg), not BSA.
• Total cumulative dosage above 550 mg/m² in adults, 300 mg/m² in children older than age 2, or 10 mg/kg in children younger than age 2 may cause myocardial toxicity.
• Dilute each 20 mg with 4 ml sterile water for injection. Further dilute each dose with 10 to 15 ml normal saline solution.
• Inject into tubing or sidearm of rapidly flowing I.V. infusion of D₅W or normal saline solution.
• For infusion, dilute further with 100 ml normal saline solution.

≫ Potentially carcinogenic

• Give single dose by I.V. injection over 3 to 5 minutes or by I.V. infusion over 30 to 45 minutes.

• Therapy requires close patient observation and frequent CBC determinations. Evaluate cardiac, renal, and hepatic function before each treatment course.

• As a precaution, allopurinol administration usually begins before antileukemic therapy starts.

• Bone marrow depression occurs in all patients given therapeutic doses. Do not start drug in patients with preexisting drug-induced bone marrow depression unless benefit warrants risk.

---

denileukin diftitox ⊠
Ontak

Indications and dosages
➡ Persistent or recurrent cutaneous T-cell lymphoma in which cancer cells express CD25 component of IL-2 receptor
Adults: 9 or 18 mcg/kg I.V. daily for 5 consecutive days, repeated every 21 days

Off-label uses (selected)

➡ Chronic lymphocytic leukemia with CD25 expression, non-Hodgkin's lymphoma
➡ Steroid-refractory graft-versus-host disease

Special considerations
• Follow hazardous drug guidelines for preparation and administration.

• Delay administration until serum albumin level reaches at least 3 g/dl.

• Before giving drug, cancer cells should be tested for CD25 expression.

• Obtain CBC, blood chemistry panel, and serum albumin levels before and weekly during therapy.

• For each 1 ml of drug from vial, add no more than 9 ml sterile saline solution without preservative to I.V. bag. Infuse over at least 15 minutes.

• Give prepared solution within 6 hours.

• During infusion, observe closely for hypersensitivity reaction. Keep appropriate drugs and resuscitative equipment at hand.

• If infusion reaction occurs, discontinue drug or reduce infusion rate.

• Evaluate patient for vascular leak syndrome, marked by at least two of

---

⊠ FDA black-box warning

following: edema, hypotension, and hypoalbuminemia. Monitor weight, edema, blood pressure, and serum albumin levels carefully.

• Monitor patients carefully for infection; cutaneous T-cell lymphoma predisposes patients to cutaneous infection.

• Loss of visual acuity, usually with or without pigment mottling, has occurred.

dexamethasone

Adrenocot, Cortastat, Cortastat LA, Cortastat 10, Dalalone, Dalalone D.P., Dalalone L.A., Decadron, Decadron 5-12 Pak, Decaject, De-Sone LA, Dexacen-4, Dexamethasone Intensol, Dexasone, Dexasone LA, Dexpak Taperpak, Hexadrol, Hexadrol Phosphate, Solurex, Solurex LA

dexamethasone acetate

dexamethasone sodium phosphate

AK-Dex, Decadron Phosphate

Indications and dosages

➡ Palliative management of leukemia and lymphoma
Adults: Dosage varies and must be individualized.
➡ Palliative management of acute leukemia
Children age 12 and older: Dosage varies with drug regimen, response, comorbidities, and other factors.
➡ Palliative management of cerebral edema associated with primary or metastatic brain tumor
Adults: 10 mg I.V. (phosphate) followed by 4 mg every 6 hours I.M. until cerebral edema symptoms subside

OFF-LABEL USES (SELECTED)

➡ Prostatic carcinoma (second-line treatment)
➡ Multiple myeloma (before bone marrow transplantation)
➡ Multiple myeloma (after bone marrow transplantation)
➡ Primary brain tumor (treatment adjunct)
➡ Fever secondary to cancer
➡ Antiemetic in cancer chemotherapy (prophylaxis for acute nausea and vomiting)

➡➡ Potentially carcinogenic

➥ Antiemetic in cancer chemotherapy (prophylaxis for delayed nausea and vomiting)
➥ Antiemetic in radiation therapy for cancer

Special considerations

• Dosage may need to be increased during stress in patients receiving long-term dexamethasone therapy.
• For primary brain tumor, dosage of 10 mg P.O. every 6 hours is commonly used but provides no antineoplastic activity. Use lowest dosage that controls symptoms.
• Drug may be given with meals and antacids between meals to prevent peptic ulcer.
• Give I.M. when oral therapy is not feasible. Do not inject I.V.
• Sodium phosphate form may be given undiluted or added to D_5W or normal saline solution and administered as infusion. Give 24-mg/ml product I.V. only.
• Interpret dexamethasone suppression test results cautiously for patients receiving concomitant indomethacin, phenytoin, phenobarbital, rifampin, or ephedrine.
• Sodium phosphate injection contains sodium bisulfite, which may cause allergic-type reactions.
• To minimize drug-induced adrenocortical insufficiency from too-rapid drug withdrawal, reduce dosage gradually.
• Carefully monitor growth and development of infants and children on prolonged therapy.

diphenhydramine hydrochloride
Banaril, Benadryl, Diphedryl, Dytan, Hyrexin, Q-Dryl, Trux-Adryl, Valu-Dryl

Indications

OFF-LABEL USES (SELECTED)

➥ Premedication for cytotoxic agents
➥ Nausea or vomiting

Special considerations

• Use injectable form only when oral forms are impractical.
• Administer I.V. at a rate of 25 mg (or fraction thereof) over 1 minute.

☒ FDA black-box warning

Extend injection time in nonemergency situations and children.
- Inject I.M. deep into large muscle mass.
- Drug is commonly combined with phenothiazine or butyrophenone to enhance antiemetic properties and reduce risk of extrapyramidal symptoms.
- Drug is more likely to cause dizziness, sedation, and hypotension in elderly patients.
- Drug may diminish mental alertness in children or cause excitation in young children.

docetaxel ⊠
Taxotere

Indications and dosages
➡ Monotherapy of locally advanced or metastatic breast cancer after chemotherapy failure
Adults: 60 to 100 mg/m^2 I.V. over 1 hour every 3 weeks; or 35 mg/m^2 I.V. infusion over 1 hour every week for 6 weeks, followed by 2-week rest period
➡ Treatment adjunct in node-positive breast carcinoma
Adults: 75 mg/m^2 I.V. 1 hour after doxorubicin 50 mg/m^2 I.V. and cyclophosphamide 500 mg/m^2 I.V. every 3 weeks for 6 courses
➡ First-line therapy in combination with cisplatin for unresectable locally advanced or metastatic non-small-cell lung cancer without previous chemotherapy
Adults: 75 mg/m^2 I.V. over 1 hour every 3 weeks
➡ Monotherapy for locally advanced or metastatic non-small-cell lung cancer after platinum-based chemotherapy failure
Adults: 75 mg/m^2 I.V. over 1 hour every 3 weeks
➡ Unresectable locally advanced or metastatic non-small-cell lung cancer in chemotherapy-naive patients, in combination with cisplatin, in patients with good performance status (ECOG 0-2)
Adults: 75 mg/m^2 I.V. over 1 hour, immediately followed by cisplatin 75 mg/m^2 I.V. over 30 to 60 minutes every 3 weeks
➡ Hormone-refractory metastatic prostate cancer, in combination with prednisone
Adults: 75 mg/m^2 I.V. over 1 hour once every 3 weeks for five to ten cycles, with prednisone 5 mg P.O. twice daily given continuously

➤➤ Potentially carcinogenic

OFF-LABEL USES (SELECTED)

➡ Small-cell lung cancer after failure of first-line chemotherapy; ovarian cancer after failure of platinum-based therapy

➡ Advanced or metastatic esophageal, gastric, or gastroesophageal junction carcinomas, including adenocarcinomas and squamous cell carcinomas

➡ Advanced, recurrent, or metastatic head and neck carcinoma, alone or in combination

➡ Bladder (urothelial) carcinoma

➡ Ovarian carcinoma after failure of platinum-based therapy

Special considerations

• Follow hazardous drug guidelines for preparation and administration.

• Adjust dosage from 100 mg/m² to 75 mg/m² in breast cancer patients who experience febrile neutropenia, neutrophil count below 500/mm³ for more than 1 week, or severe or cumulative cutaneous reactions.

• Drug should be discontinued entirely in patients who develop Grade 3 or above peripheral neuropathy.

• Withhold drug until toxicity resolves in patients with non-small-cell lung cancer receiving drug as monotherapy, patients receiving initial dosage of 75 mg/m² who experience febrile neutropenia, those with neutrophil count below 500/mm³ for more than 1 week, those with severe or cumulative cutaneous reactions, or those experiencing other Grade 3 or 4 nonhematologic toxic effects. Once symptoms resolve, drug may be resumed at dosage of 55 mg/m².

• For patients with non-small-cell lung cancer receiving combination therapy with cisplatin, if platelet-count nadir during previous course was below 25,000/mm³ or if febrile neutropenia or serious nonhematologic toxic effects occur, reduce dosage to 65 mg/m². In patients requiring further dosage reduction, 50 mg/m² is recommended.

• For patients who experience Grade 3 or 4 stomatitis, decrease dosage to 60 mg/m².

• Higher incidence of treatment-related deaths have occurred in patients with abnormal hepatic function, those receiving higher doses, and those with non-small-cell lung cancer who received previous treatment with platinum-based chemotherapy and received docetaxel as monotherapy at dosage of 100 mg/m².

• Do not give drug if patient has bilirubin level above ULN or AST or ALT level more than $1.5 \times$ ULN concomitant with ALP level above $2.5 \times$ ULN.

• To reduce severity of fluid retention and hypersensitivity reactions, premedicate all patients with oral corticosteroids.

• Reconstitute initially with diluent provided, to yield solution of 10 mg/ml. Further dilute in at least 250 ml normal saline solution or D_5W. Infuse over 1 hour.

• Perform frequent peripheral blood cell counts on all patients. Patient should not receive subsequent cycles until neutrophil count rises above $1,500/mm^3$ and platelet count rises above $100,000/mm^3$.

• Patients who respond to therapy may not show improved performance status, and may even show worsening, during therapy.

dolasetron mesylate
Anzemet

Indications and dosages
➡ Prevention of nausea and vomiting associated with initial and repeated courses of emetogenic cancer chemotherapy
Adults: 1.8 mg/kg I.V. as single dose approximately 30 minutes before chemotherapy; or fixed dose of 100 mg I.V. over 30 seconds; or 100 mg P.O. as single dose 1 hour before chemotherapy
Children ages 2 to 16: 1.8 mg/kg I.V. as single dose approximately 30 minutes before chemotherapy, to maximum of 100 mg; or 1.8 mg/kg injection solution P.O., to maximum 100-mg dose given within 1 hour before chemotherapy

OFF-LABEL USES (SELECTED)

➡ Radiation-induced nausea and vomiting

Special considerations
• Mix injection form in apple or apple-grape juice for children's oral doses.
• Single I.V. injection (up to 100 mg) may be infused over 30 seconds, or diluted in 50 ml of compatible I.V. solution (normal saline injection, D_5W injection, 5% dextrose and half-normal saline injection, 5% dextrose and lactated Ringer's injection, lactated Ringer's injection, or 10% mannitol injection) and infused over 15 minutes.

➤➤ Potentially carcinogenic

• Monitor cardiac status, especially in patients receiving other drugs that may prolong QTc interval.
• Monitor liver function tests.

---

doxorubicin hydrochloride ⊠
Adriamycin, Adriamycin PFS, Adriamycin RDF

Indications and dosages
➡ To produce regression in disseminated neoplastic conditions, such as acute lymphoblastic leukemia, acute myeloblastic leukemia, Wilms' tumor, neuroblastoma, soft-tissue and bone sarcomas, breast carcinoma, ovarian carcinoma, transitional cell bladder carcinoma, thyroid carcinoma, gastric carcinoma, Hodgkin's disease, malignant lymphoma, and bronchogenic carcinoma in which small-cell histologic type is more responsive than other cell types
Adults: As single agent, 60 to 75 mg/m^2 by slow I.V. infusion at 21-day intervals; in combination, 40 to 60 mg/m^2 by slow I.V. infusion every 21 to 28 days
➡ Ewing's sarcoma
Adults: In combination with vincristine and cyclophosphamide, alternating with ifosfamide, mesna, and etoposide, 40 to 60 mg/m^2 I.V. by slow I.V. infusion every 21 to 28 days

Off-label uses (selected)

➡ Carcinoid tumors
➡ Bladder carcinoma (prophylaxis)
➡ Primary hepatocellular carcinoma
➡ Cervical, endometrial, head, neck, pancreatic, prostatic, or testicular carcinoma; germ-cell tumors; multiple myeloma
➡ Retinoblastoma

Special considerations
⊳⊳ Follow hazardous drug guidelines for preparation and administration.
• Use lower range of recommended dosages as single I.V. injection at 21-day intervals for patients with inadequate bone marrow reserves due to old age, previous therapy, or neoplastic marrow infiltration.
• Reduce dosage in patients with hepatic impairment.

⊠ FDA black-box warning

- Drug is for I.V. use only.
- Secondary acute myelogenous leukemia has been reported.
- Consider pretreatment with allopurinol due to hyperuricemia risk.
- Reconstitute 10-, 20-, 50-, and 150-mg vials with 5, 10, 25, and 75 ml (respectively) of normal saline injection, yielding final concentration of 2 mg/ml.
- Slowly administer in tubing of free-running I.V. infusion of normal saline injection or D_5W over no less than 3 minutes.
- Local erythematous streaking along vein, as well as facial flushing, may indicate too-rapid administration.
- Stop infusion immediately and restart in another vein if patient complains of burning or stinging sensation.
- Frequently monitor CBC with differential, liver function tests, and left ventricular ejection fraction, especially as patient approaches lifetime cumulative maximum dose.
- Carefully monitor cardiac function to minimize cardiotoxicity risk.
- Acute life-threatening arrhythmias have been reported during or within a few hours after administration.
- Drug may induce tumor lysis syndrome in patients with rapidly growing tumors.
- Children are at increased risk for delayed cardiotoxicity.

doxorubicin hydrochloride, liposomal (liposomal encapsulated doxorubicin [LED]) ⊠
Doxil

Indications and dosages
➡ Metastatic ovarian carcinoma in patients with disease refractory to platinum-based chemotherapy (disease that has progressed during treatment or within 6 months of completing treatment)
Adults: 50 mg/m² (doxorubicin hydrochloride equivalent) by slow I.V. infusion at initial rate of 1 mg/minute; repeat once every 4 weeks for at least four courses as long as patient fails to progress, shows no evidence of cardiotoxicity, and continues to tolerate treatment.
➡ AIDS-related Kaposi's sarcoma in patients with disease that progressed on previous combination chemotherapy or who do not tolerate such therapy

⟫ Potentially carcinogenic

Adults: 20 mg/m² (doxorubicin hydrochloride equivalent) by slow I.V. infusion at initial rate of 1 mg/minute; repeat once every 3 weeks, for as long as patient responds satisfactorily and tolerates treatment.

OFF-LABEL USES (SELECTED)

➥ Alone or as adjunct for advanced nonovarian gynecologic cancer, solid tumors, metastatic head and neck cancer, hormone-refractory prostate cancer, glioblastoma, and metastatic brain tumor
➥ Locally advanced and metastatic breast carcinoma
➥ Multiple myeloma

Special considerations

≫ Follow hazardous drug guidelines for preparation and administration.

• Dosage adjustments may cause nonproportionally greater change in plasma level and drug exposure.

• If Grade 2 or higher adverse events occur, decrease dosage or delay therapy.

• In hepatic impairment, reduce normal dosage by 50% if serum bilirubin level is 1.2 to 3 mg/dl or by 25% if bilirubin level exceeds 3 mg/dl.

• Accidental substitution of drug for doxorubicin hydrochloride has caused severe side effects. Doxorubicin liposomal should not be substituted for conventional doxorubicin on per-mg basis.

• Consider pretreatment with allopurinol due to hyperuricemia risk.

• Patients require pretreatment with or concomitant use of antiemetics.

• Do not give drug I.M. or subcutaneously or as bolus injection or undiluted solution.

• Dilute appropriate dose (to maximum of 90 mg) in 250 ml D_5W. Do not use other diluents.

• Administer at initial rate of 1 mg/minute to help minimize risk of infusion reactions. If no infusion reaction occurs, increase rate to complete infusion over 1 hour.

• Drug is irritant (but not vesicant). Avoid extravasation.

• Monitor liver function tests and CBC with differential frequently. Carefully monitor cardiac function because severe cardiotoxicity may occur precipitously.

• Observe for signs and symptoms of palmar-plantar erythrodysesthesia, which may become severe, requiring drug withdrawal.

epirubicin hydrochloride ⊠
Ellence

Indications and dosages
➡ Adjuvant therapy in patients with evidence of axillary-node tumor involvement after resection of primary breast cancer
Adults: Initially, 100 to 120 mg/m² by I.V infusion; repeated in 3- to 4-week cycles

OFF-LABEL USES (SELECTED)

➡ Esophageal carcinoma, esophagogastric junction carcinoma, and adenocarcinoma in combination with other agents
➡ Locally unresectable and metastatic gastric carcinoma
➡ Non-small-cell lung carcinoma
➡ Limited and extensive small-cell lung carcinoma
➡ Stage III and IV (FIGO) ovarian carcinoma
➡ Hodgkin's lymphoma
➡ Non-Hodgkin's lymphoma
➡ Soft-tissue sarcoma
➡ Bladder cancer
➡ Prostate cancer
➡ Primary hepatocellular carcinoma

Special considerations
• Follow hazardous drug guidelines for preparation and administration.
• After first cycle, dosage adjustments should be based on hematologic and nonhematologic toxicities.
• Consider lower starting dosages for heavily pretreated patients, preexisting bone marrow depression, or existing neoplastic bone marrow infiltration.
• Reduce dosage in hepatic impairment; consider lower dosages in patients with severe renal impairment.
• Drug must not be given I.M. or subcutaneously.
• Secondary acute myelogenous leukemia has occurred in patients with breast cancer treated with epirubicin and other anthracyclines.
• Before initial treatment and during each cycle, perform careful baseline assessment of blood counts; serum total bilirubin, AST, and creati-

nine; and cardiac function, as well as evaluation of left ventricular ejection fraction.

• Give antiemetic before therapy begins, particularly when administering drug in conjunction with other emetogenic drugs.

• If drug is administered with paclitaxel, give paclitaxel after epirubicin.

• Do not exceed cumulative dose of 900 mg/m^2 because of cardiomyopathy risk.

• Drug is intended for I.V. infusion only (except off-label intravesicular use). Do not administer I.V. push because of risk of extravasation.

• Administer slowly into free-running I.V. infusion of normal saline solution or 5% glucose solution. Infusion should take 3 to 20 minutes.

• Immediately stop infusion and restart in another vein. Perivenous infiltration may occur without pain.

• Monitor serum uric acid, potassium, calcium phosphate, and creatinine levels immediately after initial therapy. Hydration, urine alkalization, and prophylaxis with allopurinol to prevent hyperuricemia may minimize potential complications of tumor lysis syndrome.

• Monitor patient for bone marrow depression, thrombophlebitis (including pulmonary embolism), and cardiotoxicity.

• Drug may cause inflammatory recall reaction at radiation sites.

epoetin alfa
Epogen, Procrit

Indications and dosages

➥ Anemia in patients with nonmyeloid cancers, when anemia results from effects of concomitantly administered chemotherapy; to decrease need for transfusions in patients receiving concomitant chemotherapy for at least 2 months

Adults: 150 units/kg subcutaneously three times weekly, with dosage adjusted to response after 8 weeks; or 40,000 units subcutaneously weekly, with dosage adjusted to response after 4 weeks

Off-label uses (selected)

➥ Chronic anemia associated with neoplastic disease and cancer

➥ Anemia associated with myelodysplastic syndromes (MDS) in selected patients

---

⊠ FDA black-box warning

Special considerations
• Patients with MDS commonly need higher-than-usual dosages to achieve response.
• If response is unsatisfactory, increase dosage up to 300 units/kg three times weekly or 60,000 units weekly.
• If hematocrit exceeds 40%, withhold drug until level falls to 36%.
• Administer dose slowly to decrease stinging at injection site.
• Measure hematocrit once weekly until stabilized; then measure periodically.
• Monitor patient for iron deficiency; underlying infectious, inflammatory, or malignant processes; occult blood loss; underlying hematologic disease; vitamin deficiencies; hemolysis; aluminum intoxication; and osteitis fibrosa cystica.
• Monitor blood pressure carefully.

erlotinib
Tarceva

Indications and dosages
➥ Locally advanced or metastatic non-small-cell lung cancer after failure of at least one chemotherapy regimen
Adults: 150 mg P.O. at least 1 hour before or 2 hours after food ingestion, continued until disease progression or unacceptable toxicity occurs. There is no evidence that treatment beyond progression is beneficial.
➥ First-line treatment for locally advanced, unresectable, or metastatic pancreatic cancer (with gemcitabine)
Adults: 100 mg P.O. daily at least 1 hour before or 2 hours after food ingestion, continued until disease progression or unacceptable toxicity occurs

OFF-LABEL USES (SELECTED)

➥ Colorectal and renal cell cancer
➥ Malignant glioma

Special considerations
• If patient develops acute onset of new or progressive pulmonary symptoms, withhold drug pending evaluation.
• If interstitial lung disease develops, discontinue drug.

➤➤ Potentially carcinogenic

- Administer drug at least 1 hour before or 2 hours after food ingestion.
- Periodically monitor liver function tests.
- Monitor INR and prothrombin time regularly in patients receiving warfarin, other coumarin anticoagulants, or nonsteroidal anti-inflammatory drugs.

estramustine phosphate sodium
Emcyt

Indications and dosages
➡ Palliation of metastatic or progressive prostatic cancer
Adults: 14 mg/kg P.O. in three or four divided doses with water at least 1 hour before or 2 hours after meals; continued for 30 to 90 days before deciding whether to continue therapy

OFF-LABEL USES (SELECTED)
➡ Hormone-refractory prostatic cancer

Special considerations
- Follow hazardous drug guidelines for preparation and administration.
- Give drug with water at least 1 hour before or 2 hours after meals.
- Treat patients for 30 to 90 days before determining possible benefits of continued therapy.
- Monitor patients with history of diabetes, thrombophlebitis, thrombosis, or thromboembolic disorders or with cerebrovascular or coronary artery disease.
- Drug may exacerbate preexisting or incipient peripheral edema or heart failure.
- Monitor liver function tests at appropriate intervals during therapy, and repeat 2 months after drug withdrawal.

estrogens, conjugated ☒
Premarin, Premarin Intravenous

Indications and dosages
➡ Palliation of inoperable breast cancer in appropriately selected postmenopausal women and men with metastatic disease

☒ FDA black-box warning

Adults: 10 mg P.O. three times daily for 3 months or longer
➥ Palliation of advanced androgen-dependent prostatic cancer
Adults: 1.25 to 2.5 mg P.O. three times daily

Off-label uses (selected)

➥ Salvage treatment of hemorrhagic cystitis caused by cyclophosphamide or ifosfamide

Special considerations

• Follow hazardous drug guidelines for preparation and administration.
• Patients with end-stage renal failure should receive 25% to 50% of usual dosage.
• Drug increases risk of endometrial carcinoma.
• Drug should not be used during pregnancy.
• Obtain complete medical and family history before starting therapy.
• I.V. drug is compatible with normal saline solution, dextrose, and invert sugar solutions.
• Give parenteral form by slow I.V. infusion.
• If hypercalcemia occurs, withdraw drug and take appropriate measures to reduce serum calcium level.
• Oral contraceptives may be associated with hepatic adenoma.
• Drug may trigger plasma triglyceride elevations, leading to pancreatitis and other complications.
• Large doses used to treat prostate or breast cancer are more likely to cause thrombolytic adverse reactions.
• Carefully monitor patients with diabetes mellitus or history of depression.

etoposide (VP-16) ⊠
Toposar, VePesid

etoposide phosphate ⊠
Etopophos

Indications and dosages

➥ Refractory testicular tumors in patients who have received appropriate surgical, chemotherapeutic, and radiotherapeutic therapy
Adults: In combination with other approved chemotherapeutic agents,

➤➤ Potentially carcinogenic

50 to 100 mg/m² I.V. (etoposide for injection or equivalent doses of phosphate form) daily on days 1 through 5; or 100 mg/m² I.V. daily on days 1, 3, and 5; repeated at 3- to 4-week intervals after adequate recovery from any toxicity

➥ Small-cell lung cancer as first-line treatment

Adults: In combination with other approved chemotherapeutic agents, dosage range is 35 mg/m² I.V. (etoposide for injection or equivalent doses of phosphate form) daily for 4 days to 50 mg/m² daily for 5 days, or etoposide capsules P.O. at twice the I.V. dosage and rounded to nearest 50 mg.

Off-label uses (selected)

➥ Carcinoma of unknown primary site
➥ First-line treatment of carcinoma of unknown primary site
➥ Ewing's sarcoma
➥ Hodgkin's lymphoma, high-dose chemotherapy with stem-cell rescue
➥ High-dose conditioning regimens for allogeneic bone marrow transplantation in children
➥ Bone marrow transplantation conditioning regimen for children with rhabdomyosarcoma or neuroblastoma
➥ Non-small-cell lung carcinoma
➥ Brain tumors in children
➥ Advanced neuroblastoma in children
➥ Osteosarcoma and soft-tissue sarcoma, in combination with ifosfamide and platinum
➥ Acute myelocytic leukemia in children

Special considerations

⯮ Follow hazardous drug guidelines for preparation and administration.
• Modify dosage if patient is receiving other drugs with myelosuppressive effects or has had previous radiation therapy or chemotherapy.
• If platelet count is below 50,000/mm³ or absolute neutrophil count is below 500/mm³, withhold drug until counts have sufficiently recovered.
• Reduce dosage in renal and hepatic impairment.
• Plastic devices made of acrylic or ABS may crack and leak when used with undiluted etoposide injection.
• Dilute etoposide for injection before use with D_5W or normal saline injection, for final concentration of 0.2 to 0.4 mg/ml.

• Administer solution over 30 to 60 minutes; hypotension may follow rapid I.V. administration.
• Reconstitute contents of each etoposide phosphate vial with 5 or 10 ml sterile water for injection, D_5W, normal saline injection, sterile bacteriostatic water for injection to concentration equivalent to 20 mg/ml or 10 mg/ml etoposide (22.7 mg/ml or 11.4 mg/ml etoposide phosphate), respectively.
• Administer etoposide phosphate solutions over as little as 5 minutes or up to 210 minutes.
• Monitor CBC with differential frequently, and observe for bone marrow depression during and after therapy.
• Monitor patients with low serum albumin because of increased risk of drug toxicities.

exemestane
Aromasin

Indications and dosages
➡ Advanced breast cancer in postmenopausal women whose disease progresses after tamoxifen therapy
Adults: 25 mg P.O. once daily after a meal, continued until tumor progression appears

Special considerations
• Follow hazardous drug guidelines for preparation and administration.
• For patients receiving drug with potent CYP3A4 inducer (such as rifampin or phenytoin), give 50 mg P.O. once daily after a meal.
• Monitor renal and hepatic function.
• Drug is indicated only for postmenopausal women.

filgrastim
Neupogen

Indications and dosages
➡ To decrease incidence of infection in patients with nonmyeloid cancers who are receiving myelosuppressive chemotherapy; to reduce time

to neutrophil recovery and fever duration after chemotherapy treatment of adults with acute myeloid leukemia

Adults: Initially, 5 mcg/kg subcutaneously or by I.V. infusion daily over 15 to 30 minutes, with first dose no sooner than 24 hours after chemotherapy ends; continue therapy every day for up to 2 weeks until absolute neutrophil count (ANC) reaches 10,000/mm³

➡ Neutropenia and neutropenia-related sequelae in patients with nonmyeloid cancers who are undergoing myeloablative chemotherapy followed by bone marrow transplantation

Adults: Initially, 10 mcg/kg by I.V. infusion daily over 4 or 24 hours or as continuous 24-hour subcutaneous infusion, given no sooner than 24 hours after chemotherapy and bone marrow infusion

➡ To reduce incidence and duration of neutropenia sequelae in symptomatic patients with congenital, cyclic, or idiopathic neutropenia

Adults: Initially, for patients with congenital neutropenia, 6 mcg/kg subcutaneously twice daily; for patients with cyclic or idiopathic neutropenia, 5 mcg/kg subcutaneously daily

OFF-LABEL USES (SELECTED)

➡ AIDS-associated neutropenia
➡ Myelodysplastic syndrome

Special considerations

• For myelosuppressive chemotherapy, dosage may be increased in increments of 5 mcg/kg for each cycle, according to duration and severity of ANC nadir.
• During neutrophil recovery after bone marrow transplantation, adjust daily dosage to neutrophil response.
• If necessary, drug may be diluted in D₅W.
• If drug is diluted to concentrations between 5 and 15 mcg/ml, protect from adsorption to plastic materials by adding albumin (human) to final concentration of 2 mg/ml. Do not dilute to final concentration below 5 mcg/ml.
• In patients receiving chemotherapy, monitor CBC before chemotherapy and twice weekly during chemotherapy to check for excessive leukocytosis.
• Monitor hematocrit, CBC, and platelet count at least three times weekly after bone marrow transplantation.
• Rare cases of splenic rupture (some fatal) have been reported.

floxuridine ⊠
FUDR

Indications and dosages

➥ Metastatic primary malignant neoplasm of GI tract; adenocarcinoma and secondary malignant neoplasm of liver in patients considered incurable by surgery or other means

Adults: 0.1 to 0.6 mg/kg daily by continuous arterial infusion; or 0.4 to 0.6 mg/kg daily usually by hepatic artery infusion

OFF-LABEL USES (SELECTED)

➥ Palliative management of colorectal adenocarcinoma with hepatic metastasis

➥ Ovarian carcinoma not responsive to other antimetabolites

➥ Metastatic renal carcinoma

➥ Solid tumors

Special considerations

• Follow hazardous drug guidelines for preparation and administration.

• Discontinue therapy promptly if any of these toxicity signs appears: myocardial ischemia, stomatitis or esophagopharyngitis, leukopenia or rapidly falling WBC count, intractable vomiting, diarrhea, frequent bowel movements, watery stools, GI ulceration and bleeding, thrombocytopenia, or hemorrhage from any site.

• Drug is approved for intra-arterial infusion only.

• Because severe toxic reactions may occur, all patients should be hospitalized for first course.

• Reconstitute by adding 5 ml sterile water for injection.

• Dilute intra-arterial calculated daily doses with D_5W or normal saline injection.

• Use infusion pump suitable for overcoming pressure in large arteries and ensuring uniform infusion rate.

• Carefully monitor WBC and platelet counts and renal and hepatic function.

• Drug may cause severe hematologic toxicity, GI hemorrhage, and even death despite careful patient selection and dosage adjustment.

fludarabine phosphate ☒
Fludara

Indications and dosages

➥ Refractory B-cell chronic lymphocytic leukemia after treatment with at least one standard alkylating-agent regimen

Adults: 25 mg/m^2 I.V. over 30 minutes daily for 5 consecutive days, with each 5-day cycle starting every 28 days

OFF-LABEL USES (SELECTED)

➥ Relapsed non-Hodgkin's lymphoma
➥ Acute lymphocytic leukemia in children and adults ages 1 to 21
➥ Solid tumors in children and adults ages 1 to 21

Special considerations

• Follow hazardous drug guidelines for preparation and administration.
• Reconstitute by adding 2 ml of sterile water for injection. Use within 8 hours.
• Monitor CBC and platelet counts regularly. Duration of clinically significant cytopenia ranges from approximately 2 months to 1 year.
• Drug may lead to tumor lysis syndrome.
• Monitor for excessive toxicity in patients with renal insufficiency or bone marrow impairment.

fluorouracil (5-fluorouracil, 5-FU) ☒
Adrucil, Carac, Efudex, Fluoroplex

Indications and dosages

➥ Palliative management of colon, rectum, breast, stomach, or pancreas carcinoma

Adults: Various dosing regimens

➥ Superficial basal cell carcinoma when conventional methods are impractical

Adults: 5% cream or solution topically twice daily in amount sufficient to cover lesions, continued for at least 3 to 6 weeks

Special considerations

• Follow hazardous drug guidelines for preparation and administration.

• If patient is obese or has had spurious weight gain, base dosage on estimated lean body mass, not body weight.

• Patients should be hospitalized for first course of therapy due to potential for severe toxic reactions.

• Obtain WBC count before each parenteral dose.

• Dosages given by I.V. injection do not require dilution. Administer drug by direct I.V infusion over 1 to 2 minutes.

• Drug may be diluted in normal saline solution or D_5W for continuous infusion, usually given over 24 hours.

• Topical application causes erythema, usually followed by vesiculation, erosion, ulceration, necrosis, and epithelialization.

• Use porous gauze dressing for topical form to avoid inflammatory reactions in adjacent normal skin.

• Carefully monitor patient, including CBC with differential and platelet count.

• Monitor renal and hepatic function.

• Drug can cause severe hematologic toxicity, GI hemorrhage, and death despite meticulous patient selection and careful dosage adjustment.

• Drug has been associated with palmar-plantar erythrodysesthesia. Drug withdrawal brings gradual resolution over 5 to 7 days.

• Drug may cause angina and coronary vasospasms.

---

flutamide ⊠
Eulexin

Indications and dosages

➥ Locally confined stage B2-C and stage D2 metastatic carcinoma of prostate

Adults: In combination with luteinizing hormone–releasing hormone (LH-RH) agonists, two capsules (250 mg) P.O. every 8 hours, for total daily dose of 750 mg

Special considerations

• Follow hazardous drug guidelines for preparation and administration.

• Measure serum transaminase levels before treatment, monthly for first 4 months of therapy, and then periodically.

- Capsule may be opened and contents mixed with soft food, such as applesauce or pudding.
- Carefully monitor PT in patients also receiving warfarin.
- Closely monitor liver function test results.
- Drug is highly protein-bound and is not cleared by hemodialysis.
- For patient with objective disease progression and elevated prostate-specific antigen (PSA) level, consider initiating treatment-free period of antiandrogen while continuing LH-RH.
- Breast cancer has been reported in men treated with drug.
- Discontinue flutamide if patient has evidence of clinical or PSA progression when receiving this combination, while maintaining castrate testosterone levels with either LH-RH agonist analogues or orchiectomy.

fulvestrant
Faslodex

Indications and dosages
➡ Hormone receptor–positive metastatic breast cancer in postmenopausal women with disease progression after antiestrogen therapy
Adults: 250 mg I.M. monthly as single 5-ml injection or two concurrent 2.5-ml injections

Special considerations
- Follow hazardous drug guidelines for preparation and administration.
- Administer I.M. injection slowly into large muscle (gluteal).
- Do not give subcutaneously, I.V., or intra-arterially.
- Obtain estrogen receptor assay before starting therapy.
- Monitor liver function tests and blood chemistries and plasma lipids.

gefitinib ⊠
Iressa

Indications and dosages
➡ Locally advanced or metastatic non-small-cell lung cancer after failure of platinum-based and docetaxel chemotherapies
Adults: 250 mg P.O. daily

⊠ FDA black-box warning

Special considerations

- If patient experiences acute onset or worsening of pulmonary symptoms, stop drug and initiate appropriate treatment.
- For patients receiving potent CYP3A4 inducers (such as rifampin or phenytoin), consider increasing dosage to 500 mg daily in absence of severe adverse reactions.
- Do not crush or break film-coated tablet. Tablets can be dispersed only in half-glass of noncarbonated drinking water. Have patient drink immediately.
- Monitor INR or prothrombin time regularly in patients receiving warfarin.
- Observe closely for interstitial lung disease; incidence is 1%, with one-third of cases fatal.

gemcitabine hydrochloride
Gemzar

Indications and dosages

➡ Locally advanced (nonresectable Stage II or III) or metastatic (Stage IV) adenocarcinoma of pancreas in patients previously treated with flu-orouracil

Adults: 1,000 mg/m^2 I.V. over 30 minutes once weekly for up to 7 weeks, followed by 1 week without treatment; subsequent cycles of weekly infusions for 3 consecutive weeks out of every 4 weeks

➡ Inoperable locally advanced (Stage IIIA or IIIB) or metastatic (Stage IV) non-small-cell lung cancer

Adults: In combination with cisplatin, 1,000 mg/m^2 I.V. over 30 minutes on days 1, 8, and 15 of 28-day cycle, with cisplatin 100 mg/m^2 I.V. given on day 1 after gemcitabine infusion; or 1,250 mg/m^2 I.V. over 30 minutes on days 1 and 8 of 21-day cycle, with cisplatin 100 mg/m^2 I.V. given on day 1 after gemcitabine infusion

➡ Breast cancer

Adults: In combination with paclitaxel, 1,250 mg/m^2 I.V. over 30 minutes on days 1 and 8 of each 21-day cycle, with paclitaxel 175 mg/m^2 given before gemcitabine on day 1 of each cycle

⏩ Potentially carcinogenic

OFF-LABEL USES (SELECTED)

➠ Locally advanced, unresectable, or metastatic gallbladder carcinomas or biliary tract carcinomas (such as cholangiocarcinoma, biliary tree carcinoma, or bile duct carcinoma)

➠ Metastatic bladder (urothelial) carcinoma

➠ Advanced or relapsed epithelial ovarian carcinoma

➠ Hodgkin's and non-Hodgkin's lymphomas

➠ Relapsed, refractory, progressive, metastatic, or nonseminomatous gonadal cancer (including testicular and ovarian cancer) and extragonadal germ cell tumor

Special considerations

• Follow hazardous drug guidelines for preparation and administration.

• Dosage may be increased by 25% in patients who complete entire cycle of therapy, provided that absolute granulocyte count and platelet nadirs exceed $1,500 \times 10^6$/L and $100,000 \times 10^6$/L, respectively, and non-hematologic toxicity has not exceeded WHO Grade 1.

• *Pancreatic cancer treatment:* If bone marrow depression occurs, therapy should be modified or suspended based on degree of toxicity.

• *Non-small-cell lung cancer treatment:* Patients may require dosage adjustments for hematologic toxicity for both gemcitabine and cisplatin.

• *Breast cancer treatment:* Dosage adjustments for hematologic toxicity are based on granulocyte and platelet counts obtained on day 8 of therapy. If bone marrow depression occurs, dosage should be modified.

• Monitor CBC with differential and platelet count before each dose and throughout therapy.

• Reconstitute by adding 5 ml normal saline solution injection to 200-mg vial or 25 ml normal saline solution injection to 1-g vial. Do not reconstitute at concentrations above 40 mg/ml.

• Give drug as prepared or dilute further with normal saline solution injection to concentration as low as 0.1 mg/ml. Infuse over 30 minutes.

• Evaluate renal and hepatic function before each dose and periodically afterward.

• Monitor patient for bone marrow depression.

• Monitor serum creatinine, potassium, calcium, and magnesium levels in patients receiving combination therapy with cisplatin.

gemtuzumab ozogamicin ⊠
Mylotarg

Indications and dosages
➡ CD33-positive acute myeloid leukemia in patients ages 60 and older who are not considered candidates for other cytotoxic chemotherapy
Adults: 9 mg/m² I.V. infusion over 2 hours; repeated 14 days later

Special considerations
- Follow hazardous drug guidelines for preparation and administration.
- Drug is for I.V. use only. Use only as a single agent.
- Drug may cause severe bone marrow depression when used at recommended doses.
- Drug can cause severe hypersensitivity reactions and other infusion-related reactions.
- Because patients with high peripheral blast counts may be at greater risk for pulmonary events and tumor lysis syndrome, consider leuko-reduction with hydroxyurea or leukapheresis to reduce peripheral WBC count below 30,000/mm³ before starting therapy.
- Reassess liver function studies before second dose.
- Do not administer as I.V. push or bolus.
- Reconstitute vial contents with 5 ml sterile water for injection, yielding 1 mg/ml. Dilute by injecting into 100-ml I.V. bag of normal saline solution injection.
- Infuse reconstituted solution over 2 hours through separate peripheral or central I.V. line.
- Interrupt infusion if patient experiences dyspnea or clinically significant hypotension.
- In most cases, infusion-related symptoms occur during or within 24 hours of infusion. To reduce incidence of such reactions, give diphenhydramine 50 mg P.O. and acetaminophen 650 to 1,000 mg P.O. 1 hour before therapy. Thereafter, give acetaminophen 650 to 1,000 mg P.O every 4 hours as needed, for two doses. Steroids also may be given before infusion.
- Monitor vital signs during infusion and for 4 hours afterward.
- Closely monitor electrolytes, CBC and platelet counts, and liver function test results.

▶▶ Potentially carcinogenic

• Monitor patients for signs and symptoms of hepatotoxicity. Deaths from hepatic failure and veno-occlusive disease have occurred.

---

goserelin acetate
Zoladex

Indications and dosages

➡ Palliative treatment of advanced prostate carcinoma
Adults: 3.6 mg subcutaneously into upper abdominal wall every 28 days; or 10.8 mg subcutaneously into upper abdominal wall every 12 weeks

➡ Treatment of locally confined Stage T2b to T4 (Stage B2-C) prostate carcinoma (in combination with flutamide and radiotherapy)
Adults: Starting 8 weeks before and continuing during radiotherapy, goserelin 3.6 mg subcutaneously with flutamide; followed in 28 days by goserelin 10.8 mg subcutaneously. Alternatively, four injections of 3.6 mg subcutaneously can be administered at 28-day intervals as two depots preceding and two during radiotherapy.

➡ Palliative treatment of advanced breast cancer
Adults: 3.6 mg subcutaneously into upper abdominal wall every 28 days

Special considerations

• Follow hazardous drug guidelines for preparation and administration.
• For palliative treatment of advanced breast cancer, dosage may be increased to 7.2 mg every 4 weeks if serum estradiol level does not fall to postmenopausal level after 8 weeks of therapy.
• In obese patients, AUC decreases by 1% to 2.5% with 1-kg weight increase.
• Local anesthetic may be used to reduce injection discomfort.
• Goserelin syringe cannot be used for aspiration.
• Follow manufacturer's instructions for syringe use and special injection technique.
• Although rare, hypersensitivity reactions have been reported.
• Drug is alternative when orchiectomy or estrogen therapy is not indicated or unacceptable to patient.
• Watch for transient worsening of symptoms, symptoms of increased testosterone level in men or increased estrogen level in women, and symptoms of worsening prostate or breast cancer.

⊠ FDA black-box warning

• Monitor testosterone level closely in obese patients who have not responded clinically to 10.8-mg dose.
• Drug may reduce bone mineral density, which may be partly irreversible.
• Ureteral obstruction and spinal cord compression may occur in patients with prostate cancer. Hypercalcemia may occur in patients with metastatic prostate or breast cancer.

granisetron hydrochloride
Kytril

Indications and dosages
➡ Prevention of nausea and vomiting associated with emetogenic cancer therapy
Adults: For oral dosing only on chemotherapy days—With 2-mg once-daily regimen, give two 1-mg tablets or 10 ml of oral solution (2 tsp, equivalent to 2 mg granisetron) up to 1 hour before chemotherapy. With 1-mg twice-daily regimen, give first 1-mg tablet or 1 tsp (5 ml) of oral solution up to 1 hour before chemotherapy, and give second tablet or second tsp (5 ml) of oral solution 12 hours after first.
Adults and children older than age 2: 10 mcg/kg I.V. within 30 minutes before start of chemotherapy and only on chemotherapy days
➡ Nausea and vomiting associated with radiation, including total body irradiation and fractionated abdominal radiation
Adults: 2 mg P.O. daily within 1 hour of radiation

Special considerations
• Injection solution may be given I.V. undiluted over 30 seconds or diluted with normal saline solution or D_5W and infused over 5 minutes.
• Prepare I.V. infusion just before administering. Dilute in normal saline solution or D_5W.
• Monitor liver function and CBC with differential.
• When given to patients with chemotherapy-induced nausea and vomiting, drug may mask progressive ileus or gastric distention.

⏩ Potentially carcinogenic

histrelin acetate implant
Vantas

Indications and dosages
➥ Palliative treatment of advanced prostate cancer
Adults: One implant subcutaneously in inner aspect of upper arm every 12 months to provide continuous drug release for 12 months

Special considerations
• Adhere to insertion and removal procedures supplied with implant.
• Insert implant subcutaneously into inner aspect of upper arm.
• Implant is not radiopaque. If it is difficult to locate by palpation, use ultrasound or CT scan.
• Monitor serum testosterone and prostate-specific antigen levels.
• Ureteral or bladder-outlet obstruction and spinal cord compression may occur and contribute to paralysis, with or without fatal complications.
• Drug causes transient testosterone increase during first week of therapy.

hydroxyurea ☒
Droxia, Hydrea, Mylocel

Indications and dosages
➥ Melanoma and recurrent, metastatic, or inoperable ovarian carcinoma
Adults: 80 mg/kg P.O. every 3 days or 20 to 30 mg/kg P.O. every day
➥ Local control of primary squamous cell (epidermoid) carcinomas of head and neck, excluding lips
Adults: In combination with radiation therapy, 80 mg/kg P.O. as single dose every 3 days beginning 7 days before start of radiation; then continuing during and after radiation therapy
➥ Resistant, chronic myelocytic leukemia
Adults: 20 to 30 mg/kg P.O. daily

Special considerations

▸▸ Follow hazardous drug guidelines for preparation and administration.

• In patients with renal impairment, dosage should be decreased up to 50% for creatinine clearance of 10 to 50 ml/minute, and up to 75% for creatinine clearance below 10 ml/minute.

• If WBC count falls below 2,500/mm^3 or platelet count drops below 100,000/mm^3, interrupt therapy until values rise significantly toward normal.

• If blood counts are within toxic range, discontinue drug until hematologic recovery occurs.

• If patient develops hematologic toxicity twice on specific dosage, do not use same dosage again.

• Capsules may be opened and mixed in water.

• Administer prophylactic folic acid as indicated.

• Keep patient hydrated (10 to 12 glasses of water daily).

• Closely monitor blood counts and kidney and liver function tests before and during therapy; obtain hemoglobin and total WBC and platelet counts as least once weekly and obtain bone marrow examination as indicated.

• Manage severe anemia with whole blood replacement without stopping hydroxyurea therapy.

• Neutropenia is usually first and most common indicator of hematologic suppression.

ibritumomab tiuxetan ⊠
In-111 Zevalin, Y-90 Zevalin

Indications and dosages

➡ Relapsed or refractory low-grade, follicular, or transformed B-cell non-Hodgkin's lymphoma, including patients with rituximab-refractory follicular non-Hodgkin's lymphoma

Adults: Therapy requires two steps. *Step 1:* Single I.V. infusion of rituximab 250 mg/m^2, followed by In-111 Zevalin 5.0 mCi (1.6 mg total antibody dose) I.V. *Step 2:* After 7 to 9 days, second I.V. infusion of rituximab 250 mg/m^2 given before Y-90 Zevalin 0.4 mCi/kg I.V.

Special considerations

• Follow hazardous drug guidelines for preparation and administration.
• Y-90 Zevalin dosage should be reduced to 0.3 mCi/kg (11.1 MBq/kg) in patients with baseline platelet count of 100,000 to 149,000/mm³.
• In-111 Zevalin and Y-90 Zevalin are not available in Zevalin kits. Isotopes must be ordered from separate manufacturers at same time that ibritumomab tiuxetan kits are ordered.
• Do not mix any regimen component with other drugs.
• Administer ibritumomab tiuxetan in the recommended two-step process.
• Observe for signs and symptoms of severe infusion reaction, such as hypotension, angioedema, hypoxia, and bronchospasm, which may require administration interruption.
• Monitor for thrombocytopenia and neutropenia.
• Monitor CBC and platelet count weekly after regimen ends, and continue until levels recover. Continue monitoring for cytopenias for up to 3 months after therapy ends.
• Although solid-organ toxicity has not been attributed to radiation from adjacent tumors, consider this potential before treating patients with very high tumor uptake next to critical organs or structures.
• Regimen results in significant radiation dose to testes.
• Drug contains human albumin, posing remote risk of viral disease transmission.

idarubicin hydrochloride ⊠
Idamycin PFS

Indications and dosages

➡ Acute myeloid leukemia in adults
Adults: Initially, 12 mg/m² daily by slow I.V. injection over 10 to 15 minutes for 3 days in combination with cytarabine. Cytarabine may be given as 100 mg/m² continuous I.V. infusion daily for 7 days, or as 25 mg/m² I.V. bolus followed by cytarabine 200 mg/m² by continuous I.V. infusion daily for 5 days. Repeat once, depending on initial response.

OFF-LABEL USES (SELECTED)

➡ Acute lymphocytic leukemia
➡ Advanced breast cancer

⊠ FDA black-box warning

Special considerations

• Follow hazardous drug guidelines for preparation and administration.
• For patients with hepatic impairment and bilirubin level of 2.6 to 5 mg/dl, dosage should be reduced by 50%.
• Drug should not be given if bilirubin level exceeds 5 mg/dl.
• For patients with renal impairment and serum creatinine level below 2.5 mg/dl, dosage decrease should be considered.
• If second course of therapy is indicated, course should be delayed in patients who experienced severe mucositis after first course, until recovery occurs; then dosage should be reduced by 25%.
• Monitor serum bilirubin and creatinine levels closely before and during therapy.
• Maximum lifetime dose is 150 mg/m^2.
• Reconstitute 20-mg powder vials with 20 ml sterile water for injection to yield final concentration of 1 mg/ml.
• Administer I.V. slowly over 10 to 15 minutes in infusion of normal saline solution injection or D_5W injection.
• Drug may induce hyperuricemia. Take appropriate steps to prevent hyperuricemia and control systemic infections before starting therapy.
• Monitor patient closely for severe bone marrow depression, which occurs in all patients receiving drug—typically within 10 to 15 days of initial dose. Obtain frequent CBC and platelets counts.
• Monitor patient for cardiotoxicity and treat appropriately.

ifosfamide ⊠
Ifex, Ifex/Mesnex

Indications and dosages

➡ Second-line chemotherapy for germ-cell testicular cancer
Adults: 1.2 g/m^2 I.V. infusion daily for 5 consecutive days; repeated every 3 weeks or after recovery from hematologic toxicity (platelet count at or above 100,000/mm^3 and WBC count at or above 4,000/mm^3); typically in combination with vinblastine and cisplatin and administered with mesna or other prophylactic agent for hemorrhagic cystitis

OFF-LABEL USES (SELECTED)

➡ Ewing's and soft-tissue sarcoma
➡ Hodgkin's and non-Hodgkin's lymphoma

⊠ Potentially carcinogenic

➥ Non-small-cell lung cancer

➥ Head and neck carcinoma; breast, cervical, endometrial, or ovarian epithelial and germ-cell carcinoma; neuroblastoma; osteosarcoma; acute lymphocytic lymphoma; bladder carcinoma; relapsed or refractory thymoma and thymic carcinoma

Special considerations

• Follow hazardous drug guidelines for preparation and administration.

• Drug has been given to patients with compromised hepatic and renal function, although optimal dosing schedules have not been determined.

• If patient experiences urotoxic adverse effects (particularly hemorrhagic cystitis) or CNS toxicities (such as confusion and coma), therapy may need to be discontinued.

• Obtain urinalysis before each dose and regularly throughout therapy. If results show microscopic hematuria with more than 10 RBCs/high-power field, withhold therapy until hematuria resolves.

• Obtain hemoglobin level and WBC and platelet counts before each dose and at appropriate intervals.

• To prevent bladder toxicity, hydrate patient with at least 2 L of oral or I.V. fluid daily.

• Administer uroprotectant such as mesna to prevent hemorrhagic cystitis.

• Reconstitute by adding 20 ml sterile water for injection or bacteriostatic water for injection.

• Solution may be diluted further in D_5W injection, normal saline solution injection, Lactated ringer's injection, or sterile water for injection.

• Administer as slow I.V. infusion over at least 30 minutes.

• Drug may cause somnolence, confusion, hallucinations and, in some cases, coma. Discontinue therapy if these occur.

• Hematuria incidence and severity can be significantly reduced through vigorous hydration, fractionated dosing schedule, and use of protector (such as mesna).

• Drug may interfere with normal wound healing.

• In patients on warfarin, monitor prothrombin time and INR closely for 3 to 4 days during initiation and withdrawal of therapy.

imatinib mesylate
Gleevec

Indications and dosages

➡ Initial treatment of Ph+ chronic myeloid leukemia (CML) in chronic phase
Adults: 400 to 600 mg P.O. daily

➡ Ph+ CML in blast crisis, accelerated phase, or chronic phase after failure of interferon alfa therapy
Adults: For chronic phase, 400 mg P.O. daily; for blast crisis or accelerated phase, 600 mg P.O. daily

➡ Kit (CD117)-positive, unresectable or metastatic malignant GI stromal tumor
Adults: 400 to 600 mg P.O. daily

➡ Recurrent Ph+ CML in chronic phase after stem cell transplant, or patients resistant to interferon alfa therapy
Children older than age 3: 260 mg/m^2 P.O. daily (tablets only)

OFF-LABEL USES (SELECTED)

➡ Acute lymphocytic leukemia, glioma, refractory prostate cancer, small-cell lung cancer, soft-tissue sarcoma

Special considerations

• Follow hazardous drug guidelines for preparation and administration.
• Dosage increase from 400 to 600 mg may be considered in patients with chronic-phase CML, or from 600 to 800 mg (400 mg twice daily) in adults in accelerated phase or blast crisis.
• For children with chronic-phase CML, increased daily dosages may be considered (under circumstances similar to those for adults in chronic phase) from 260 to 340 mg/m^2 daily, as clinically indicated.
• Increase dosage by at least 50% in patients receiving drug with potent CYP3A4 inducer (such as rifampin or phenytoin).
• For adults, if elevation in bilirubin level is above 3 × institutional upper limit of normal (IULN) or liver transaminase levels are above 5 × IULN, withhold drug until level drops.
• Reduce dosage or interrupt therapy in patients with severe neutropenia and thrombocytopenia.

➤➤ Potentially carcinogenic

• If patient experiences severe nonhematologic adverse reactions, withhold drug until event resolves.

• Monitor liver function (transaminases, bilirubin, and ALP) before therapy begins and then monthly.

• Administer with meal and large glass of water.

• In adults, give daily doses above 600 mg in two divided doses. In children, give daily doses above 400 mg in two divided doses (one in morning and one in evening).

• Obtain CBC weekly for first month, biweekly for second month, and periodically thereafter as clinically indicated.

• Cytopenia occurs more often in patients with accelerated-phase CML or blast crisis than in those with chronic-phase CML.

• Do not give warfarin. Patients requiring anticoagulation should receive low-molecular-weight or standard heparin.

• Weigh patient regularly and monitor for signs and symptoms of fluid retention, which may be severe. Higher doses increase edema risk.

• Monitor patient for GI bleeding.

• Drug may cause liver and kidney toxicities and increased rate of opportunistic infections.

• Patients taking total daily dosage of 1,200 mg may have increased iron levels and require treatment to lower iron exposure.

interferon alfa-2a, recombinant (IFLrA, rIFN-A) ☒
Roferon-A

Indications and dosages

➡ Hairy cell leukemia

Adults: For induction, 3 million international units subcutaneously daily for 16 to 24 weeks. For maintenance, 3 million international units I.M. or subcutaneously three times weekly. Dosages above 3 million international units are not recommended.

➡ Chronic myelogenous leukemia (Philadelphia-chromosome positive)

Adults: Initially, 9 million international units subcutaneously daily. Short-term tolerance may improve by gradually increasing dosage over

---

first week from 3 million international units daily for 3 days to 6 million international units daily for 3 days, to target dosage of 9 million international units daily for duration of therapy.

Children: 2.5 to 5 million international units/m^2 subcutaneously daily

OFF-LABEL USES (SELECTED)

➥ Renal-cell carcinoma
➥ Carcinoid tumors
➥ Cutaneous T-cell lymphoma
➥ Non-Hodgkin's lymphoma (low and intermediate grades)

Special considerations

• Follow hazardous drug guidelines for preparation and administration.
• If severe reactions occur in patients with Kaposi's sarcoma or hairy cell leukemia, dosage should be reduced by 50% or drug stopped temporarily until reactions abate.
• Ensure that patient is well hydrated to reduce risk of hypotension associated with fluid depletion.
• Drug is indicated for subcutaneous use only.
• Avoid using different brands in single-treatment regimen; dosage and adverse reactions vary.
• Swirl vial gently to dissolve drug.
• Monitor CBC with differential, hemoglobin, platelets, blood chemistries, hairy cells, and bone marrow hairy cells at baseline and periodically during therapy.
• In patients with Kaposi's sarcoma, obtain indicator lesion measurements and total lesion count at baseline and then monthly.
• Monitor patient closely for depression; consider stopping drug if it occurs.
• Monitor periodic liver function tests.
• Monitor ECG before and during therapy in patients with advanced cancer or preexisting cardiac disease.
• Interferon-alphas have been associated with serious or fatal GI hemorrhage.

interferon alfa-2b, recombinant (IFN-alfa 2) ⊠
Intron A

Indications and dosages
➥ Hairy cell leukemia
Adults: 2 million international units/m^2 I.M. or subcutaneously three times weekly for up to 6 months. Responding patients may benefit from continued treatment.
➥ Adjuvant to surgical treatment for malignant melanoma in patients who are free of disease but at increased risk of systemic recurrence within 56 days of treatment
Adults: 20 million international units/m^2 by I.V. infusion over 20 minutes for 5 consecutive days per week for 4 weeks, followed by maintenance dosage of 10 million international units/m^2 subcutaneously three times weekly for 48 weeks
➥ Clinically aggressive follicular non-Hodgkin's lymphoma
Adults: 5 million international units subcutaneously three times weekly for up to 18 months with anthracycline-containing chemotherapy regimen
➥ AIDS-related Kaposi's sarcoma
Adults: 30 million international units/m^2 subcutaneously or I.M three times weekly until severe intolerance or maximum response has occurred after 16 weeks of therapy. (For this indication, only 50-million international units strength should be used.)

OFF-LABEL USES (SELECTED)

➥ Renal-cell carcinoma
➥ Chronic myelogenous leukemia
➥ Follicular non-Hodgkin's lymphoma

Special considerations
• Follow hazardous drug guidelines for preparation and administration.
• *For patients with hairy cell leukemia:* If severe adverse reactions develop, interrupt therapy until reactions abate; then restart therapy at 50% of initial dosage.
• *For patients with malignant melanoma:* Discontinue drug temporarily if granulocyte count falls below 500/mm^3 or if ALT or AST level rises

above 5 to 10 × ULN. When adverse reactions abate, restart at 50% of previous dosage.

• *For patients with follicular lymphoma:* Modify regimen for evidence of serious toxicity. Delay chemotherapy regimen if neutrophil count is below 1,500/mm³ or platelet count is below 75,000/mm³.

• *For patients with AIDS-related Kaposi's sarcoma:* For severe adverse reactions, decrease dosage by 50% or stop drug temporarily until adverse reactions abate.

• Ensure that patient is well hydrated to reduce risk of hypotension.

• Do not use different brands in single treatment regimen.

• Drug is indicated as adjunctive therapy within 56 days of surgery for patients with malignant melanoma who are disease-free but at high risk for systemic recurrence. It is not intended for induction-phase treatment of malignant melanoma.

• Use multidose pens for subcutaneous injection only.

• Do not use solution for injection for I.V. administration.

• Do not use 50-million international unit strength powder for injection to treat hairy cell leukemia or follicular lymphoma.

• Do not use multidose pens or multidose vials of solution for injection to treat AIDS-related Kaposi's sarcoma.

• Do not give by I.M. injection to patients with platelet counts below 50,000/mm³.

• Antipyretics may be used to prevent or relieve fever and headache.

• Monitor CBC with differential, platelets, blood chemistries, electrolytes, liver function tests, and TSH at baseline and periodically during therapy.

• Perform baseline eye examination.

• If evidence of pulmonary infiltrates or pulmonary impairment appears, consider discontinuing therapy; monitor patient closely.

• Monitor ECG in patients with cardiovascular conditions or advanced cancer.

• Monitor patient closely for depression; consider stopping drug if depression occurs.

• Hepatotoxicity (including death) has occurred in patients receiving injection form. Closely monitor patient who develops hepatic function abnormalities during treatment.

• Diabetic patients may require adjustment of antidiabetic regimen.

>> Potentially carcinogenic

• If triglyceride level rises, provide clinically appropriate management. Consider discontinuing drug in patients with triglyceride level persistently above 1,000 mg/dl who develop pancreatitis.
• With higher dosages, obtundation and coma may occur.

---

interferon alfa-n3 (human leukocyte-derived)
Alferon N

Indications

Off-label uses (selected)

➡ Hairy cell leukemia, AIDS-related Kaposi's sarcoma, bladder carcinoma, renal carcinoma, chronic myelocytic leukemia, non-Hodgkin's lymphoma, malignant melanoma, multiple myeloma, mycosis fungoides, carcinoid tumors, epithelial ovarian carcinoma

Special considerations

• Follow hazardous drug guidelines for preparation and administration.
• Ensure that patient is well hydrated to reduce risk of hypotension.
• If patient has acute, serious hypersensitivity reaction, stop drug at once and begin appropriate medical therapy.
• Monitor CBC with differential.
• Product is made from human blood and may pose risk of transmitting viruses and other infectious agents.

---

irinotecan hydrochloride ☒
Camptosar

Indications and dosages

➡ First-line therapy with leucovorin and 5-fluorouracil (5-FU) for patients with metastatic carcinoma of colon or rectum
Adults: Administer as I.V. infusion over 90 minutes. For all regimens, give leucovorin immediately after irinotecan, and give 5-FU immediately after leucovorin. Recommended irinotecan dosages and modifications for both combination and single-agent therapy vary due to selected regimen and patient condition.
➡ Metastatic carcinoma of colon or rectum in patients whose disease

---

☒ FDA black-box warning

has recurred or progressed after initial fluorouracil-based therapy

Adults: Single-dose regimen by I.V. infusion once weekly for 4 weeks, followed by 2-week rest period. After adequate recovery, repeat additional doses in similar 6-week cycle; continue indefinitely in patients who achieve response or whose disease remains stable.

OFF-LABEL USES (SELECTED)

➥ Non-small-cell lung cancer
➥ Cervical cancer
➥ Ovarian cancer
➥ Pancreatic cancer
➥ Brain tumors
➥ Gastric cancer

Special considerations

• Follow hazardous drug guidelines for preparation and administration.
• Patients age 70 and older should receive starting dosage of 300 mg/m^2 in single-agent, once-every-3-week regimen.
• All dosage modifications should be based on worst preceding toxicity.
• Administering drug to patients with bilirubin level above 2 mg/dl is not recommended.
• Patient should be premedicated with antiemetics.
• Consider prophylactic or therapeutic administration of atropine in patients with cholinergic symptoms.
• Dilute for infusion with 250 to 500 ml D$_5$W to yield 0.12 to 2.8 mg/ml.
• Do not add other drugs to infusion solution.
• Administer by I.V. infusion. Take care to avoid extravasation. If extravasation occurs, flush site with sterile water and apply ice.
• Before each dose, carefully monitor WBC count with differential, hemoglobin, and platelets.
• Carefully monitor patient with diarrhea. Give fluid and electrolyte replacement for dehydration; give antibiotics for ileus, fever, or severe neutropenia. If Grade 2, 3, or 4 late diarrhea occurs, decrease subsequent dosages within current cycle.
• Deaths from sepsis after severe neutropenia have occurred.
• Monitor hepatic function. Patients with modestly elevated baseline serum total bilirubin levels (1 to 2 mg/dl) are at significantly greater risk for first-cycle Grade 3 or 4 neutropenia.

≫ Potentially carcinogenic

• Closely monitor patients with history of pelvic or abdominal irradiation because of increased risk of myelosuppression.

• Drug may cause colitis complicated by ulceration, bleeding, ileus, and infection. Provide prompt antibiotic support to patients with ileus.

isotretinoin (13-*cis*-retinoic acid) ⊠
Accutane, Amnesteem, Claravis, Sotret

Indications

OFF-LABEL USES (SELECTED)

➥ Squamous-cell cancer of head and neck

➥ Advanced, refractory lymphoid malignancies (given with interferon alfa)

➥ Cutaneous T-cell lymphoma

Special considerations

• Dosage should be adjusted based on disease response or appearance of adverse effects.

• Isotretinoin must be prescribed under iPLEDGE program.

• Female patients must have had two negative pregnancy tests with a sensitivity of at least 25 mIU/ml before receiving drug.

• Obtain pretreatment liver function tests and blood lipid levels under fasting conditions.

• Administer drug with meal.

• Repeat pregnancy test monthly before patient receives each prescription.

• Monitor WBC count for neutropenia.

• Obtain follow-up blood lipid levels under fasting conditions.

• Obtain follow-up liver function tests at weekly or biweekly intervals until response to drug is established.

• Monitor patient carefully for vision problems. If these occur, stop drug and make sure patient receives ophthalmologic examination.

• Accutane may cause hearing impairment, which may persist even after therapy ends.

• Closely monitor blood glucose and serum CK levels.

⊠ FDA black-box warning

• Acute pancreatitis may occur in patients with elevated or normal serum triglyceride levels. Stop Accutane if hypertriglyceridemia cannot be controlled at acceptable level or if pancreatitis symptoms occur.

lenalidomide ⊠
Revlimid

Indications and dosages
➡ Transfusion-dependent anemia resulting from low- or intermediate-1-risk myelodysplastic syndrome associated with deletion 5q cytogenic abnormality (with or without additional cytogenic abnormalities)
Adults: 10 mg P.O. daily

Special considerations
• Follow hazardous drug guidelines for preparation and administration.
• If thrombocytopenia develops within 4 weeks of starting treatment at 10 mg daily, adjust dosage as necessary based on platelet counts.
• If neutropenia develops after 4 weeks of starting treatment at daily dosage of 10 mg, interrupt treatment if neutrophil count falls below 500/mm^3 for approximately 7 days, or falls below 500/mm^3 associated with fever of approximately 101.3° F (38.5° C).
• Drug is analogous of thalidomide, a known teratogen that causes severe, life-threatening birth defects.
• Drug may be prescribed only by licensed prescribers registered in RevAssist program and may be obtained only through controlled distribution program through contracted pharmacy.
• Before drug is prescribed, female patient should have had two negative pregnancy tests with a sensitivity of at least 50 mIU/ml.
• First pregnancy test should be done within 10 to 14 days before prescribing, second test within 24 hours before prescribing, and then regularly during therapy..
• Monitor CBC weekly for first 8 weeks, and then at least monthly.
• Observe carefully for signs and symptoms of thromboembolism.
• Patient must be able to reliably follow instructions to take drug and must be informed about conditions of RevAssist program.

letrozole
Femara

Indications and dosages
➡ First-line treatment of hormone-receptor-positive or hormone-receptor-unknown locally advanced or metastatic breast cancer in postmenopausal women; treatment of advanced breast cancer in postmenopausal women with disease progression after antiestrogen therapy; adjuvant treatment of postmenopausal women with hormone-receptor-positive early breast cancer; extended adjuvant treatment of early breast cancer in postmenopausal women who have received 5 years of adjuvant tamoxifen therapy
Adults: 2.5-mg tablet P.O. once daily without regard to meals

OFF-LABEL USES (SELECTED)
➡ Prevention of recurrence of early-stage breast cancer and prevention of new breast cancer (based on studies using anastrozole)

Special considerations
• Follow hazardous drug guidelines for preparation and administration.
• In patients with cirrhosis or severe hepatic impairment, dosage should be reduced to 50% of usual dosage.
• Dosage reduction is recommended in patients with creatinine clearance of 10 ml/minute or less.
• Continue therapy until tumor progression occurs.
• Patients do not require glucocorticoid or mineralocorticoid replacement during therapy.
• Monitor hepatic and renal function.

leuprolide acetate
Eligard, Lupron, Lupron Depot, Viadur

Indications and dosages
➡ Advanced prostate cancer
Adults: Injection—1 mg daily subcutaneously. *Depot*—7.5 mg I.M. monthly, 22.5 mg I.M. every 3 months, or 30 mg I.M. every 4 months. *Implant*—72 mg subcutaneously once yearly.

☒ FDA black-box warning

➡ Treatment of breast cancer
➡ Treatment of endometrial cancer
➡ Treatment of ovarian cancer

Special considerations

• Follow hazardous drug guidelines for preparation and administration.
• Patients with known allergies to benzyl alcohol may experience symptoms of hypersensitivity.
• Shake vial well to achieve uniform suspension. Withdraw entire contents of single-use vial into syringe and inject immediately.
• Depot form does not contain preservative.
• Preexisting hematuria and urinary tract obstruction has temporarily worsened during first week of therapy. Also, a few cases of temporary weakness and paresthesia of lower limbs have occurred.
• With implant, serum testosterone level increases transiently during first week. Patient may experience new or worsening symptoms, including bone pain, neuropathy, hematuria, or ureteral or bladder outlet obstruction.
• Bone density loss may be irreversible for 6 months or more.
• In patients with prostate cancer, monitor response by measuring serum testosterone and acid phosphatase levels.
• Monitor response 1 to 2 months after therapy begins with gonadotropin-releasing hormone stimulation test and sex steroid levels.
• In therapeutic dosages, depot suppresses pituitary-gonadal system. Normal function usually resumes within 1 to 3 months after treatment ends.
• Diagnostic tests of pituitary gonadotropic and gonadal functions may be misleading during therapy and for up to 1 to 2 months afterward.

lomustine ⊠
CeeNU

Indications and dosages

➡ Brain tumors (both primary and metastatic) in patients who have undergone appropriate surgical or radiotherapeutic procedures; secondary therapy with other approved drugs in patients with Hodgkin's

⟫ Potentially carcinogenic

disease who relapse during primary therapy or fail to respond to primary therapy

Adults and children: As single agent in previously untreated patients, 130 mg/m^2 P.O. as a single dose every 6 weeks. Do not give repeat course of capsules until circulating blood elements return to acceptable levels (platelet count above 100,000/mm^3 and WBC count above 4,000/mm^3), which usually occurs in 6 weeks. Peripheral blood smear should show adequate number of neutrophils.

OFF-LABEL USES (SELECTED)

➥ Melanoma, multiple myeloma, breast cancer, non-small-cell lung cancer, colorectal cancer
➥ Non-Hodgkin's lymphoma
➥ Kidney cancer
➥ Mycosis fungoides

Special considerations

〉〉 Follow hazardous drug guidelines for preparation and administration.

• In compromised bone marrow function, reduce dosage to 100 mg/m^2 every 6 weeks.
• Most adverse reactions are reversible if detected early.
• When giving capsules with other myelosuppressants, adjust dosage accordingly.
• After initial dose, adjust subsequent dosages based on hematologic response to preceding dose.
• Obtain CBC and platelet counts before starting therapy.
• Give drug on empty stomach, preferably 2 to 4 hours after meal.
• Administer antiemetics as needed.
• Myelosuppression usually occurs 4 to 6 weeks after therapy ends and is dose-related. Thrombocytopenia occurs about 4 weeks after therapy and lasts 1 to 2 weeks. Leukopenia arises 5 to 6 weeks after therapy and lasts 1 to 2 weeks.
• Monitor blood counts weekly. Do not give repeat courses before 6 weeks because hematologic toxicity is delayed and cumulative.
• Although rare, pulmonary toxicity may occur with capsule use.
• Monitor liver and renal function tests periodically.

lorazepam
Ativan, Lorazepam Intensol

Indications and dosages
➡ Anxiety disorders, short-term relief of symptoms of anxiety or anxiety associated with depressive symptoms
Adults: Usual dosage is 2 to 6 mg daily P.O. in divided doses, not to exceed 10 mg daily. (Daily dosage may vary from 1 to 10 mg.)
Elderly adults: 1 to 2 mg daily P.O. in divided doses
Children: 0.05 mg/kg P.O. every 4 to 8 hours

Off-label uses (selected)
➡ Chemotherapy-induced nausea and vomiting

Special considerations
• To avoid oversedation in elderly or debilitated patients, do not exceed initial daily dosage of 2 mg, and increase gradually according to patient's response.
• Monitor patient and adjust dosage in renal or hepatic impairment.
• Administer largest dose at bedtime.
• When giving drug I.M., inject undiluted deep into muscle mass.
• Sublingual dose absorbs faster than P.O. dose, with effect comparable to that of I.M. dose.
• Immediately before I.V. administration, dilute injection form with equal volume of compatible solution. Inject directly into vein or tubing of existing I.V. infusion at a rate no faster than 2 mg/minute.
• Drug may cause leukopenia or low-density lipoprotein elevations. Obtain periodic CBC with differential and liver function tests in patients on long-term therapy.
• Monitor vital signs and cardiovascular and respiratory function.
• Patients should be monitored for signs and symptoms of upper GI disease when drug is used for prolonged periods or in elderly patients.
• Monitor for paradoxical reactions, especially in elderly patients and children.
• Prolonged use may cause dependence. Withdrawal may occur after 4 to 6 weeks.

➡➡ Potentially carcinogenic

mechlorethamine hydrochloride (HN_2, nitrogen mustard) ☒
Mustargen

Indications and dosages

➡ Palliative treatment of Hodgkin's disease (stages III and IV), lymphosarcoma, chronic myelocytic or chronic lymphocytic leukemia, polycythemia vera, mycosis fungoides, and bronchogenic carcinoma
Adults: Dosage varies with clinical situation, therapeutic response, and magnitude of hematologic depression. Total dosage of 0.4 mg/kg for each course usually is given either as single dose or in divided doses of 0.1 to 0.2 mg/kg daily I.V.

➡ Palliative treatment of metastatic carcinoma resulting in effusion
Adults: For intracavitary injection, usual dosage is 0.4 mg/kg. Dosage of 0.2 mg/kg (or 10 to 20 mg) has been given by intrapericardial route.

Off-label uses (selected)

➡ Cutaneous T-cell lymphoma

Special considerations

⪢ Follow hazardous drug guidelines for preparation and administration.

- Base dosage on ideal dry body weight.
- Drug is a powerful vesicant intended mainly for I.V. use.
- Before giving drug, obtain accurate histologic diagnosis of patient's disease, knowledge of its natural course, and adequate clinical history; also evaluate hematologic status.
- Use care in dosing; drug has narrow margin of safety.
- Administer at night in case patient requires sedation for adverse effects.
- Administer with antiemetics.
- Concomitant use with sedatives may be beneficial.
- Ensure adequate fluid intake before treatment begins to help control hyperuricemia.
- Using sterile 10-ml syringe, inject 10 ml sterile water for injection or 10 ml sodium chloride injection into vial.
- To administer I.V., withdraw into syringe the calculated solution volume needed for a single injection. Although drug may be injected di-

☒ FDA black-box warning

rectly into any suitable vein, injecting it into rubber or plastic tubing of flowing I.V. infusion set is preferable and reduces risk of severe local reactions.

• Give total dose I.V. over 3 to 5 minutes.
• Technique and dosage for intracavitary route vary.
• Lymphocytopenia usually occurs within 24 hours of administration. Granulocytopenia and thrombocytopenia usually occur 6 to 8 days after dose, and last 10 days to 3 weeks. Agranulocytopenia is rare. Leukopenia generally resolves by 2 weeks.
• Do not give subsequent courses until patient recovers hematologically from previous course.
• Do not give drug before or after radiation therapy until bone marrow function recovers.
• Give drug with extreme caution to patients with chronic lymphatic leukemia.
• Bone and nervous tissue tumors respond poorly to drug.
• Drug should not be used routinely in patients with widely disseminated neoplasms.
• Hyperuricemia may develop during therapy. Anticipate urate precipitation. Institute adequate methods for controlling hyperuricemia.
• Drug has caused many hepatic and renal abnormalities in patients with neoplastic disease.
• Drug may be associated with increased incidence of secondary cancer.
• Drug has caused extensive and rapid development of amyloidosis.
• Nausea and vomiting typically begin 1 to 3 hours after dose.
• Intracavitary route is indicated for patients with pleural, peritoneal, or pericardial effusion caused by metastatic tumors.
• Death has been reported after intracavitary administration. Avoid intracavitary route when patient is receiving systemic therapy with other agents that may suppress bone marrow function.

medroxyprogesterone acetate ⊠
Amen, Curretab, Cycrin, Depo-Provera, Provera

Indications and dosages
➡ Adjunctive therapy and palliative treatment of inoperable, recurrent, or metastatic endometrial or renal carcinoma
Adults: Initially, 400 to 1,000 mg I.M. weekly; if improvement occurs

and disease appears to be stabilized, it may be possible to maintain improvement with as little as 400 mg per month.

OFF-LABEL USES (SELECTED)

➟ Advanced breast cancer

Special considerations

• Perform breast and pelvic examination and Papanicolaou test as pretreatment evaluation.

• Inject drug deeply into deltoid or gluteal muscle.

• Be alert to earliest manifestations of thrombotic disorders. Stop drug promptly if these occur or are suspected.

• Stop drug (pending examination) if patient experiences sudden partial or complete vision loss or sudden onset of proptosis, diplopia, or migraine. If examination shows papilledema or retinal vascular lesions, withdraw drug.

• Stop drug if signs or symptoms of hepatic impairment occur.

• Monitor liver function tests, glucose and thyroid-stimulating hormone levels, and coagulation tests.

• Evaluate patient for signs and symptoms of thrombotic disorders.

• Drug may exacerbate signs and symptoms of depression.

---

megestrol acetate ☒
Megace, Megace ES

Indications and dosages

➟ Palliative treatment of advanced breast carcinoma (recurrent, inoperable, or metastatic)
Adults: 40 mg P.O. four times daily (tablets) for at least 2 months
➟ Palliative treatment of endometrial carcinoma (recurrent, inoperable, or metastatic)
Adults: 40 to 320 mg P.O. daily (tablets) in divided doses for at least 2 months

OFF-LABEL USES (SELECTED)

➟ Ovarian adenocarcinoma and related gynecologic cancers (high-dose megestrol)
➟ Advanced breast cancer (high-dose megestrol)

☒ FDA black-box warning

➡ Prostate cancer
➡ Cancer-related anorexia and cachexia

Special considerations

• Follow hazardous drug guidelines for preparation and administration.
• Risk of toxic reactions may be greater in patients with renal impairment.
• Use of tablets during first 4 months of pregnancy is not recommended. If patient is exposed to drug during first 4 months of pregnancy or becomes pregnant during therapy, inform her of potential risks to fetus.
• Pretreatment evaluation in women should include breast and pelvic examinations and Papanicolaou test.
• Give drug with food to decrease adverse GI effects.
• Monitor hematologic tests, thyroid-stimulating hormone level, and coagulation tests.
• In elderly patients, monitor liver and kidney function tests.
• Drug may exacerbate diabetes mellitus and increase insulin requirements. Monitor serum glucose level.
• Closely monitor patients with history of thromboembolic disease.
• Consider risk of adrenal insufficiency during prolonged therapy or withdrawal from prolonged therapy in patients with signs or symptoms of hypoadrenalism. Failure to recognize hypothalamic-pituitary-adrenal inhibition may result in death.

melphalan (L-PAM) ⊠
Alkeran, Alkeran I.V.

Indications and dosages

➡ Palliative treatment of multiple myeloma in patients for whom oral therapy is not appropriate
Adults: 16 mg/m² I.V. as single infusion over 15 to 20 minutes; given at 2-week intervals for four doses and then, after adequate recovery from toxicity, at 4-week intervals
➡ Palliative treatment of multiple myeloma
Adults: 6 mg (three tablets) P.O. daily. Entire daily dose may be given at one time. Adjust dosage, as needed, based on blood counts at intervals of approximately 1 week. After 2 to 3 weeks, stop drug for up to 4 weeks; during this hiatus, follow blood counts carefully. When WBC

➡➡ Potentially carcinogenic

and platelets counts are rising, give maintenance dosage of 2 mg daily. Because of patient variations in drug plasma levels with P.O. use, escalate dosage cautiously until some myelosuppression occurs, to ensure that potentially therapeutic drug levels have been reached.

OFF-LABEL USES (SELECTED)

➡ Bone marrow transplantation in non-Hodgkin's lymphoma

Special considerations

➤➤ Follow hazardous drug guidelines for preparation and administration.

• Consider dosage reduction of up to 50% in patients with renal insufficiency (BUN at least 30 mg/dl) who are receiving drug I.V.

• Consider dosage adjustment based on blood counts at nadir and on treatment day.

• Repeated courses or continuous therapy should be given because improvement may continue slowly over many months.

• Hypersensitivity reactions (including anaphylaxis) have occurred in about 2% of patients who received drug I.V.

• Obtain at least one CBC with differential before each dose.

• Give oral dose on empty stomach to enhance absorption.

• Reconstitute drug for injection by rapidly injecting 10 ml of supplied diluent (yields 5 mg/ml solution) directly into vial of lyophilized powder using 20G or larger needle.

• Immediately dilute dose in normal saline solution injection to a concentration no greater than 0.45 mg/ml.

• Give diluted product over at least 15 minutes. Complete administration within 60 minutes of reconstitution.

• Monitor hematologic function with weekly CBC count with differential throughout therapy. Observe patient closely for signs and symptoms of bone marrow depression.

• If WBC count is below 3,000/mm^3 or platelet count is below 100,000/mm^3, stop drug until counts recover.

• Giving prednisone with drug may enhance palliation of multiple myeloma symptoms.

• Secondary cancers have occurred in cancer patients receiving drug.

mercaptopurine ⊠
Purinethol

Indications and dosages

➡ Acute lymphatic (lymphocytic, lymphoblastic) leukemia (ALL), acute myelogenous and acute myelomonocytic leukemia

Adults and children: Dosage is calculated to nearest multiple of 25 mg. Total daily dosage may be given at one time. Therapy consists of two steps—induction and maintenance. *Induction:* Dosage is individualized. Initiate with 2.5 mg/kg P.O. daily (100 to 200 mg in average adult, 50 mg in average 5-year-old child). If no clinical improvement and no definite evidence of WBC or platelet depression occur after 4 weeks at this dosage, increase up to 5 mg/kg daily. *Maintenance:* Once complete hematologic remission occurs, maintenance therapy is essential. Usual maintenance dosage is 1.5 to 2.5 mg/kg P.O. daily as single dose.

Special considerations

- Follow hazardous drug guidelines for preparation and administration.
- Consider dosage reduction in patients with renal or hepatic impairment.
- Stop drug temporarily at first sign of abnormally steep decrease in WBC count, platelet count, or hemoglobin.
- Patients with inherited thiopurine methyltransferase deficiency may be unusually sensitive to drug's myelosuppressive effects and may develop rapid bone marrow suppression after initial therapy. To avoid life-threatening marrow suppression, dosage must be reduced substantially.
- Reduce dosage when drug is given concomitantly with xanthine oxidase inhibitor.
- Studies in children with ALL suggest that administering drug in evening reduces risk of relapse.
- Evaluate hemoglobin or hematocrit, total WBC count with differential, and quantitative platelet count weekly during therapy.
- Monitor liver function tests weekly when therapy begins and monthly thereafter. More frequent testing may be needed in patients who are receiving other hepatotoxic drugs or have preexisting hepatic disease. If patient develops jaundice, hepatomegaly, or anorexia with right hypochondrium tenderness, withdraw drug immediately until exact cause is determined.

➡➡ Potentially carcinogenic

- When given as single agent for induction, drug induces complete remission in about 25% of children and 10% of adults.
- Drug is not effective in CNS leukemia, chronic lymphocytic leukemia, lymphomas (including Hodgkin's), and solid tumors.
- Drug may cause subnormal response to infectious agents or vaccines.
- Drug rarely should be relied on as single agent for maintaining remission in acute leukemia.

mesna
Mesnex

Indications and dosages

➡ Prophylaxis to reduce incidence of ifosfamide-induced hemorrhagic cystitis

Adults: Mesna may be given on fractionated dosing schedule of three bolus I.V. injections or as single bolus injection followed by two oral administrations of mesna tablets as described below. If patient vomits within 2 hours of oral mesna dose, repeat dose or administer drug by I.V. route.

I.V. dosing schedule

Mesna is given as I.V. bolus injections in dosage equal to 20% of ifosfamide dosage (weight/weight) at time of ifosfamide administration and 4 and 8 hours after each ifosfamide dose. Total daily mesna dosage is 60% of ifosfamide dosage. See recommended dosing schedule below.

Drug	0 hours	2 hours	6 hours
ifosfamide	1.2 g/m^2	None	None
mesna	240 mg/m^2	240 mg/m^2	240 mg/m^2

I.V. and P.O. dosing schedule

Mesna injection is given as I.V. bolus injections in dosage equal to 20% of ifosfamide dosage (weight/weight) at time of ifosfamide administration. Mesna tablets are given P.O. in dosage equal to 40% of ifosfamide dosage 2 and 6 hours after each ifosfamide dose. Total daily mesna dosage is 100% of ifosfamide dosage. See the following recommended dosing schedule.

Drug	0 hours	2 hours	6 hours
ifosfamide	1.2 g/m²	None	None
mesna	240 mg/m²	480 mg/m²	480 mg/m²

OFF-LABEL USES (SELECTED)

➡ Prophylaxis to reduce incidence of cyclophosphamide-induced hemorrhagic cystitis

➡ Cyclophosphamide-induced hemorrhagic cystitis in bone marrow transplant recipients

Special considerations

• Dosing schedule should be repeated on each day that ifosfamide is administered. When ifosfamide dosage is adjusted (either increased or decreased), mesna-to-ifosfamide ratio should be maintained.

• For I.V. administration, drug can be diluted (for final concentration of 20 mg mesna/ml) in any of the following fluids: 5% dextrose injection, 5% dextrose and 0.45% sodium chloride injection, 0.92% sodium chloride injection, or lactated Ringer's injection.

• Give I.V. bolus over 1 minute.

• Drug does not inhibit ifosfamide-induced adverse reactions other than hemorrhagic cystitis.

• Patients with autoimmune disorders who receive mesna and cyclophosphamide may have higher incidence of allergic reactions.

methotrexate sodium ⊠
Rheumatrex Dose Pack, Trexall

Indications and dosages

➡ Gestational choriocarcinoma, chorioadenoma destruens, hydatidiform mole

Adults: 15 to 30 mg P.O. or I.M. daily for 5-day course; repeat three to five times as needed, with rest periods of 1 week or more interposed between courses until manifesting toxic symptoms subside

➡ Acute lymphoblastic leukemia

Adults and children: To induce remission, 3.3 mg/m² daily with 60 mg/

m^2 prednisone. For maintenance, twice weekly P.O. or I.M. in total weekly doses of 30 mg/m^2, or 2.5 mg/kg I.V. every 14 days.

➥ Meningeal leukemia (therapeutic and preventive)

Children age 3 and older: 12 mg preservative-free form intrathecally every 2 to 5 days

Children age 2: 10 mg preservative-free form intrathecally every 2 to 5 days

Children age 1: 8 mg preservative-free form intrathecally every 2 to 5 days

Children younger than age 1: 6 mg preservative-free form intrathecally every 2 to 5 days

➥ Burkitt's lymphoma

Adults: For stages I and II, 10 to 25 mg P.O. daily for 4 to 8 days; for stage III, 0.625 to 2.5 mg/kg P.O. daily with other antitumor agents, interposed with 7- to 10-day rest periods

➥ Breast cancer, epidermoid cancers of head and neck, advanced mycosis fungoides (cutaneous T-cell lymphoma), lung cancer (especially squamous-cell and small-cell types)

Adults: Various regimens have been used.

➥ Mycosis fungoides (cutaneous T-cell lymphoma)

Adults: Methrotrexate 5 to 50 mg once weekly, or 15 to 37.5 mg twice weekly in patients who respond poorly to weekly therapy. Combination chemotherapy regimens that include methotrexate I.V. at higher doses with leucovorin rescue have been used in advanced disease stages.

➥ Lymphosarcoma (stage III)

Adults: 0.625 mg/kg to 2.5 mg/kg P.O. daily

➥ Nonmetastatic osteosarcoma in patients who have undergone surgical resection or amputation for primary tumor

Adults: Methrotrexate 12 g/m^2 I.V. as 4-hour infusion in weeks 4, 5, 6, 7, 11, 12, 15, 16, 29, 30, 44, and 44 after surgery. Give in combination with leucovorin 15 mg P.O. every 6 hours for 10 doses beginning 24 hours after start of methotrexate infusion, in addition to combinations of other chemotherapeutic agents (which may include doxorubicin, cisplatin, and bleomycin-cyclophosphamide-dactinomycin [BCD] regimen). If dosage does not produce peak serum methotrexate concentration of 1,000 μM (10^{-3} mol/L) at end of methotrexate infusion, dosage may be increased to 15 g/m^2 in subsequent treatments.

⊠ FDA black-box warning

OFF-LABEL USES (SELECTED)

➥ Bladder cancer
➥ Head and neck cancer

Special considerations

• Follow hazardous drug guidelines for preparation and administration.
• Drug is given until CSF cell count returns to normal, at which time additional dose is recommended.
• As appropriate, adjust, reduce, or discontinue systemic antileukemic therapy based on neurologic adverse reactions.
• Most adverse reactions are reversible if detected early. When these occur, reduce dosage or stop therapy and take appropriate corrective measures.
• In patients with renal impairment, ascites, or pleural effusions, reduce dosage or, in some cases, withdraw drug.
• Interrupt drug therapy for diarrhea and ulcerative stomatitis; otherwise, hemorrhagic enteritis and death from intestinal perforation may occur.
• Malignant lymphomas may occur in patients receiving low doses and may not require cytotoxic treatment. Discontinue drug first; if lymphoma does not regress, begin appropriate treatment.
• Drug may induce tumor lysis syndrome in patients with rapidly growing tumors.
• Severe and occasionally fatal skin reactions have occurred after single or multiple doses.
• Potentially fatal opportunistic infections may occur.
• When given concomitantly with radiotherapy, drug may increase risk of soft-tissue necrosis and osteonecrosis.
• Perform baseline assessment, including CBC with differential and platelet count, hepatic enzyme levels, renal function tests, and chest X-ray.
• Oral administration of tablet form is often preferred when low dosages are given because of rapid absorption and effective serum levels.
• Methotrexate isotonic liquid for injection and powder for injection may be given by I.M., I.V., intra-arterial, or intrathecal route.
• Reconstitute each vial with preservative-free D_5W or normal saline solution; 25 mg/ml is maximum concentration that can be given I.V. Further dilute single dose with D_5W or normal saline solution immediately before infusing higher doses (100 mg or more).

➤➤ Potentially carcinogenic

- For I.V. injection, give each 10 mg over 1 minute. For I.V. infusion, give each dose over 30 minutes to 4 hours.
- For intrathecal use, dilute preservative-free drug to concentration of 1 mg/ml in appropriate sterile, preservative-free medium (such as normal saline solution injection). CSF volume depends on age, not body surface area.
- With high-dose therapy, follow safety guidelines for leucovorin rescue. If patient vomits or cannot tolerate oral medication, give leucovorin I.V. or I.M. at same dosage and on same schedule.
- Drug clearance rate varies widely and generally decreases at higher doses.
- Frequently monitor CBC with differential, platelet count, liver enzyme levels, renal function tests, and chest X-ray during initiation of therapy, after dosage changes, or during periods of increased risk of elevated methotrexate blood level (such as dehydration).
- Promptly evaluate patient with profound granulocytopenia and fever.
- Monitor patient for acute chemical arachnoiditis.
- Chronic leukoencephalopathy manifests as confusion, irritability, somnolence, ataxia, dementia, seizures, and coma. This condition can be progressive and even fatal.
- Monitor for transient acute neurologic syndrome, which may occur with high-dose regimens.
- Monitor for subacute myelopathy characterized by paraparesis or paraplegia associated with involvement of one or more spinal nerve roots.
- Pulmonary symptoms or nonspecific pneumonitis may indicate potentially dangerous lesion and warrant therapy interruption and careful investigation.
- High doses used in osteosarcoma treatment may cause renal damage, leading to acute renal failure. Monitor renal function closely. Monitor serum drug and creatinine levels.
- Transient liver function test abnormalities are common after methotrexate administration and rarely necessitate modification of methotrexate therapy.
- In women with childbearing potential, do not start methotrexate until pregnancy has been excluded.

mitomycin ⊠
Mutamycin

Indications and dosages

➡ Disseminated adenocarcinoma of stomach or pancreas in combination with other chemotherapeutic agents, or as palliative treatment when other modalities have failed

Adults or adolescents: After full hematologic recovery from previous chemotherapy, 20 mg/m² I.V. as single dose at 6- to 8-week intervals

Off-label uses (selected)

➡ Bladder cancer
➡ Squamous-cell cancer of anus (combination therapy)

Special considerations

》 Follow hazardous drug guidelines for preparation and administration.

• For patients with WBC count below 2,000/mm³ and platelet count below 25,000/mm³, give 50% of previous dose.

• When giving drug with other myelosuppressants, adjust dosage.

• Do not give drug to patients with serum creatinine above 1.7 mg/dl.

• Systemic therapy may cause hemolytic uremic syndrome (HUS). HUS may occur at any time when drug is used as single agent or in combination with other cytotoxic drugs. However, most cases occur at dosage of at least 60 mg. Blood transfusion may exacerbate HUS symptoms.

• Drug may cause acute shortness of breath and severe bronchospasm, with symptom onset occurring within minutes to hours of injection.

• To dilute 5-mg, 20-mg, and 40-mg vials, add 10 ml, 40 ml, or 80 ml sterile water for injection, respectively. May dilute further for infusion with D_5W injection, normal saline solution, or sodium lactate injection.

• Administer single dose by I.V. injection over 5 to 10 minutes; infusion rate depends on amount and type of solution.

• Adult respiratory distress syndrome has occurred in several patients receiving drug with other chemotherapeutic agents who were maintained on fraction of inspired oxygen above 50% preoperatively. Administer only enough oxygen for adequate arterial saturation. Monitor fluid balance carefully, avoiding overhydration.

》 Potentially carcinogenic

• Drug causes high incidence of bone marrow depression. Obtain repeated studies of platelets, WBC with differential, and hemoglobin during therapy.
• Observe patient for signs and symptoms of renal toxicity.

mitotane ⊠
Lysodren

Indications and dosages
➡ Inoperable adrenocortical carcinoma
Adults: 2 to 6 g P.O. daily in three to four divided doses, increased incrementally to 9 or 10 g daily P.O. in divided doses. Maximum daily dosage is 19 g.

Special considerations
• Follow hazardous drug guidelines for preparation and administration.
• If severe side effects occur, reduce dosage to maximum tolerated amount.
• Dosage should be decreased in patients with hepatic disease.
• Start treatment in hospital until patient achieves stable dosage regimen.
• Some authorities recommend concomitant steroid replacement during therapy.
• If clinical benefits do not occur after 3 months at maximum tolerated dosage, consider therapy a clinical failure.
• Long-term continuous, high-dose therapy may lead to brain damage and functional impairment.
• Drug may accelerate warfarin metabolism, raising warfarin dosage requirement. Carefully monitor patient receiving warfarin or other coumarin-type anticoagulant for change in dosage requirements.

mitoxantrone hydrochloride ⊠
Novantrone

Indications and dosages
➡ Pain related to advanced hormone-refractory prostate cancer (combination therapy with corticosteroids)

⊠ FDA black-box warning

Adults: 12 to 14 mg/m² given as a short I.V. infusion every 21 days

➤ Initial treatment of acute nonlymphocytic leukemia (ANLL) in combination with other approved drugs

Adults: For induction, 12 mg/m² I.V. infusion daily on days 1 to 3, with 100 mg/m² cytarabine given as continuous 24-hour infusion daily on days 1 to 7. In incomplete antileukemic response to initial course, second induction course may be given for 2 days and cytarabine may be given for 5 days at same daily dosages after all signs or symptoms of severe or life-threatening nonhematologic toxicity have resolved.

Off-label uses (selected)

➤ Breast cancer

➤ Non-Hodgkin's lymphoma

➤ Chronic myelocytic leukemia in blast phase, nonlymphocytic leukemia

Special considerations

》》 Follow hazardous drug guidelines for preparation and administration.

• Except in ANLL treatment, drug generally should not be given to patients with baseline neutrophil counts below 1,500/mm³.

• Before each dose, left ventricular ejection fraction (LVEF) evaluation by echocardiogram or MUGA scan is recommended. Do not give drug if LVEF is below 50% or if significant reduction occurs.

• Monitor CBC with platelet count before each course and if signs or symptoms of infection develop. Monitor liver function tests before each course.

• Treat systemic infections concomitantly with or just before therapy begins.

• Dilute dose to at least 50 ml with normal saline solution injection or D_5W injection. Drug may be diluted further in D_5W, normal saline solution, or dextrose 5% with normal saline solution. Use immediately.

• Do not mix in same infusion with other drugs. Introduce diluted solution slowly into tubing as free-running I.V. infusion over 3 to 5 minutes.

• When given in high doses (above 14 mg/m² daily for 3 days), drug may cause severe myelosuppression.

• Observe patient closely for signs and symptoms of infection and bleeding.

》》 Potentially carcinogenic

• Occasionally, acute congestive heart failure occurs in patients receiving drug for ANLL.

• Monitor uric acid level. Maintain hydration, provide hypouricemic therapy, and alkalize urine if necessary.

---

nilutamide ☒
Nilandron

Indications and dosages

➥ Metastatic prostate cancer

Adults: 300 mg P.O. once daily for 30 days; then 150 mg P.O. once daily

Special considerations

• Follow hazardous drug guidelines for preparation and administration.

• At onset of dyspnea or worsening of preexisting dyspnea, interrupt drug therapy and determine if respiratory symptoms are drug-related. If findings suggest interstitial pneumonitis, stop drug.

• Before starting drug, obtain baseline liver enzyme levels and routine chest X-ray.

• Drug can be taken with or without food.

• For greatest benefit, start therapy on day of or after orchiectomy.

• Monitor liver enzymes at regular intervals (every 3 months); if transaminases increase more than 2 to 3 × ULN, stop drug.

• Perform appropriate laboratory tests at first sign or symptom of hepatic injury (such as jaundice, dark urine, fatigue, abdominal pain, and unexplained GI symptoms).

---

oxaliplatin ☒
Eloxatin

Indications and dosages

➥ Advanced carcinoma of colon or rectum (combination therapy with infusional fluorouracil [5-FU]) and leucovorin in patients whose disease has recurred or progressed during or within 6 months after completing first-line therapy with combination of 5-FU/leucovorin and irinotecan

Adults: *Day 1*—oxaliplatin 85 mg/m^2 I.V. infusion in 250 to 500 ml

---

☒ FDA black-box warning

D_5W and leucovorin 200 mg/m^2 I.V. infusion in D_5W, both given over 120 minutes at same time in separate bags using Y-line; followed by 5-FU 400 mg/m^2 I.V. bolus over 2 to 4 minutes; followed by 5-FU 600 mg/m^2 I.V. infusion in 500 ml D_5W (recommended) as 22-hour continuous infusion. *Day 2*—leucovorin 200 mg/m^2 I.V. infusion over 120 minutes; followed by 5-FU 400 mg/m^2 I.V. bolus over 2 to 4 minutes; followed by 5-FU 600 mg/m^2 I.V. infusion in 500 ml D_5W (recommended) as 22-hour continuous infusion. Repeat cycle every 2 weeks.

OFF-LABEL USES (SELECTED)

➡ Non-small-cell lung cancer
➡ Esophageal cancer
➡ Ovarian cancer
➡ Head and neck cancer

Special considerations

• Follow hazardous drug guidelines for preparation and administration.
• Prolonging infusion time from 2 to 6 hours decreases peak concentration by estimated 32% and may mitigate acute toxicities.
• For patients who experience persistent Grade 2 neurosensory events that do not resolve, consider reducing oxaliplatin dosage to 65 mg/m^2. For patients with persistent Grade 3 neurosensory events, consider stopping therapy.
• Reducing oxaliplatin dosage to 65 mg/m^2 and 5-FU by 20% (300 mg/m^2 bolus and 500 mg/m^2 as 22-hour infusion) is recommended for patients after recovery from Grade 3/4 GI toxicity.
• Premedication with antiemetics is recommended.
• Do not reconstitute or dilute drug with sodium chloride solution or other chloride-containing solutions.
• Reconstitute lyophilized powder by adding 10 ml (50-mg vial) or 20 ml (100-mg vial) water for injection or D_5W injection. Further dilute with 250 to 500 ml 5% dextrose infusion solution.
• Drug is incompatible in solution with alkaline drugs or media (such as basic 5-FU solutions) and must not be mixed with these or administered simultaneously through same infusion line. Flush infusion line with D_5W before administering any concomitant drug.
• Hypersensitivity and anaphylactic or anaphylactoid reactions (rash, urticaria, erythema, pruritus and, rarely, bronchospasm and hypotension) may occur within minutes of administration. These reactions usu-

ally are managed with standard epinephrine, corticosteroids, or antihistamine therapy and may require drug discontinuation.
• Monitor I.V. site closely to avoid extravasation.
• Monitor patient closely for signs and symptoms of acute pharyngolaryngeal dysesthesia syndrome.
• Drug may cause persistent and primarily peripheral sensory neuropathy marked by paresthesia, dysesthesia, and hypoesthesia. Condition also may include proprioception deficits that interfere with daily activities.
• Watch for unexplained respiratory signs and symptoms. Discontinue drug until further pulmonary investigation excludes interstitial lung disease or pulmonary fibrosis.

paclitaxel ⊠
Onxol, Taxol

Indications and dosages
➥ Advanced carcinoma of ovary
Adults: For previously untreated patients, paclitaxel 175 mg/m² I.V. over 3 hours followed by 75 mg/m² cisplatin I.V. every 3 weeks; or paclitaxel 135 mg/m² I.V. over 24 hours followed by 75 mg/m² cisplatin I.V. every 3 weeks. For previously treated patients, paclitaxel 135 or 175 mg/m² I.V. over 3 hours every 3 weeks.
➥ Adjuvant treatment of node-positive breast cancer
Adults: 175 mg/m² I.V. over 3 hours every 3 weeks for four courses, given sequentially with combination chemotherapy that includes doxorubicin
➥ Breast cancer after failure of combination chemotherapy for metastatic disease or relapse within 6 months of adjuvant chemotherapy
Adults: 175 mg/m² I.V. over 3 hours every 3 weeks
➥ Non-small-cell lung cancer in patients ineligible for potentially curative surgery or radiation therapy
Adults: 135 mg/m² I.V. over 24 hours followed by 75 mg/m² cisplatin I.V. every 3 weeks
➥ AIDS-related Kaposi's sarcoma
Adults: 135 mg/m² I.V. over 3 hours every 3 weeks, or 100 mg/m² I.V. over 3 hours every 2 weeks

⊠ FDA black-box warning

OFF-LABEL USES (SELECTED)

➥ Head and neck cancer
➥ Metastatic esophageal cancer
➥ Prostate cancer
➥ Advanced gastric cancer

Special considerations

• Follow hazardous drug guidelines for preparation and administration.
• In patients with advanced HIV, reduce dosage of dexamethasone (as one of three premedication drugs) to 10 mg P.O. (instead of 20 mg P.O.); initiate or repeat paclitaxel therapy only if neutrophil count is at least 1,000/mm³; reduce paclitaxel dosage in subsequent courses by 20% for patients with severe neutropenia (neutrophil count below 500/mm³ for 1 week or more); and initiate concomitant hematopoietic growth factor (G-CSF), as clinically indicated.
• For patients with solid tumors, do not repeat paclitaxel course until neutrophil count is at least 1,500/mm³ and platelet count is at least 100,000/mm³.
• In patients who develop severe neutropenia (neutrophil count below 500/mm³ for 1 week or more) or severe peripheral neuropathy during therapy, reduce dosage by 20% in subsequent courses.
• Patients with hepatic impairment may be at increased risk for toxicity, particularly Grade 3-4 myelosuppression.
• Premedicate all patients to prevent severe hypersensitivity reactions.
• Before infusion, dilute drug in normal saline solution injection, D₅W injection, 5% dextrose and normal saline solution injection, or 5% dextrose in Ringer's injection to final concentration of 0.3 to 1.2 mg/ml.
• Do not use PVC containers or administration sets.
• Monitor infusion site closely for infiltration because of extravasation risk.
• Monitor blood counts frequently. Do not retreat patient with subsequent cycles until neutrophil count recovers to above 1,500/mm³ (above 1,000/mm³ for patients with Kaposi's sarcoma) and platelet count recovers to above 100,000/mm³.
• Perform continuous cardiac monitoring during subsequent therapy if patient develops significant conduction abnormalities during drug infusion.
• Monitor blood pressure and heart rate frequently.

• Drug contains dehydrated alcohol (396 mg/ml); consider possible CNS and other effects of alcohol.

---

paclitaxel protein-bound particles ⊠
Abraxane

Indications and dosages

➡ Treatment of breast cancer after failure of combination chemotherapy for metastatic disease or relapse within 6 months of adjuvant therapy; previous therapy should have included an anthracycline (unless clinically contraindicated).

Adults: 260 mg/m² I.V. over 30 minutes every 3 weeks

Special considerations

• Follow hazardous drug guidelines for preparation and administration.

• If patient experiences severe neutropenia (neutrophil count of 500/mm³ for 1 week or longer) or severe sensory neuropathy, reduce dosage in subsequent courses to 220 mg/m².

• Drug should not be administered to metastatic breast cancer patients with baseline neutrophil counts below 1,500/mm³.

• This albumin form of paclitaxel may substantially affect drug's functional properties (compared to drug in solution). Do not substitute for or with other paclitaxel formulations.

• Drug is supplied as sterile lyophilized powder for reconstitution before use. To avoid errors, read entire preparation instructions before reconstitution.

• Each milliliter of reconstituted formulation contains 5 mg/ml paclitaxel.

• To calculate exact total dosing volume of 5-mg/ml suspension required for patient, use this formula:

Dosing volume (ml) = total dose (mg)/5 (mg/ml)

• To reconstitute each vial, slowly inject 20 ml normal saline solution injection over at least 1 minute. Once injection is complete, let vial sit for at least 5 minutes to ensure proper wetting of lyophilized cake or powder. Then gently swirl or invert vial slowly for at least 2 minutes until cake or powder dissolves completely. If foaming or clumping occurs,

---

⊠ FDA black-box warning

let solution stand for at least 15 minutes until foam subsides. Do not filter.

• Obtain frequent peripheral blood counts to monitor for neutropenia and thrombocytopenia. Patient should not be retreated in subsequent cycles until neutrophil count recovers to above 1,500/mm3 and platelet count recovers to above 100,000/mm³.

palonosetron hydrochloride
Aloxi

Indications and dosages
➡ Prevention of acute nausea and vomiting associated with initial and repeat courses of moderately or highly emetogenic cancer chemotherapy; prevention of delayed nausea and vomiting associated with initial and repeat courses of moderately emetogenic chemotherapy
Adults: 0.25 mg I.V. about 30 minutes before chemotherapy starts. Do not repeat sooner than 7 days.

Special considerations
• Give drug undiluted; infuse I.V. over 30 seconds. Do not mix with other drugs. Flush infusion line with normal saline solution before and after administration.
• Monitor vital signs and ECG.
• Monitor electrolyte and blood glucose levels.

pegaspargase
Oncaspar

Indications and dosages
➡ Acute lymphoblastic leukemia in patients who require L-asparaginase but have developed hypersensitivity to native L-asparaginase forms; given in combination with other chemotherapy drugs
Adults and children with body surface area (BSA) 0.6 m² or more: 2,500 international units/m² I.M. or I.V. every 14 days
Children with BSA under 0.6 m²: 82.5 international units/kg I.M. or I.V. every 14 days

➤➤ Potentially carcinogenic

Special considerations

- Follow hazardous drug guidelines for preparation and administration.
- Drug is not recommended for use as sole induction agent.
- Avoid excessive agitation of vial. Do not shake.
- I.M. route is preferred. Limit volume at single injection site to 2 ml.
- For I.V. use, administer over 1 to 2 hours in 100 ml sodium chloride or dextrose injection 5% through already-running infusion.
- Observe patient for 1 hour after administration. Keep resuscitation equipment and appropriate drugs on hand to treat anaphylaxis.
- Obtain frequent serum amylase levels to detect early evidence of pancreatitis.
- Monitor blood glucose, fibrinogen, PT, and PTT frequently.
- When using with hepatotoxic chemotherapy, monitor patient for hepatic dysfunction.
- Observe patient closely for signs and symptoms of infection.

---

pegfilgrastim
Neulasta

Indications and dosages

➡ To reduce incidence of infection in patients with nonmyeloid malignancies who are receiving myelosuppressive anticancer drugs associated with clinically significant incidence of febrile neutropenia
Adults and children weighing more than 45 kg (99 lb): 6 mg subcutaneously once per chemotherapy cycle

Special considerations

- Drug should be discontinued or withheld until adult respiratory distress syndrome (ARDS) resolves.
- Obtain CBC and platelet count before chemotherapy begins.
- Do not give drug 14 days before or 24 hours after cytotoxic chemotherapy because rapidly dividing myeloid cells may have increased sensitivity to cytotoxic chemotherapy.
- Do not use 6-mg, fixed-dose, single-use syringe form in infants, children, or smaller adolescents weighing less than 99 lb.
- To activate UltraSafe Needle Guard, place hands behind needle, grasp guard with one hand, and slide guard forward until needle is completely covered and guard clicks into place.

⊠ FDA black-box warning

• Regularly monitor patient's hematocrit and platelet count.
• If patient has left upper abdominal or shoulder tip pain, evaluate for enlarged spleen. Rare cases of splenic rupture have occurred.
• ARDS has occurred in neutropenic patients with sepsis who have received filgrastim.

pemetrexed
Alimta

Indications and dosages

➡ Malignant pleural mesothelioma in patients whose disease is unresectable or who are not otherwise candidates for curative surgery
Adults: Pemetrexed 500 mg/m^2 I.V. infusion over 10 minutes on day 1 of each 21-day cycle, in combination with cisplatin 75 mg/m^2 infused over 2 hours starting approximately 30 minutes after pemetrexed administration ends
➡ Locally advanced or metastatic non-small-cell lung cancer after previous chemotherapy
Adults: 500 mg/m^2 I.V. infusion over 10 minutes on day 1 of each 21-day cycle

Special considerations

• For pemetrexed and cisplatin therapy–induced hematologic toxicities with nadir absolute neutrophil count (ANC) below 500/mm^3 and nadir platelet count of 50,000/mm^3 or more, give 75% of previous dosages of both drugs. For such toxicities in which nadir ANC is below 50,000/mm^3 (regardless of nadir platelet count), give 50% of previous dosages of both drugs.
• If patient develops nonhematologic toxicity (excluding neurotoxicity) at or greater than Grade 3 (except Grade 3 transaminase elevation), withhold pemetrexed until toxicity resolves to less than or equal to pre-therapy value.
• Do not administer when creatinine clearance is below 45 ml/minute.
• Drug is intended for I.V. use only.
• Pretreatment with dexamethasone reduces incidence and severity of cutaneous reactions.
• Hydrate patient (usually 1 to 2 L of fluid infused over 8 to 12 hours)

⟫ Potentially carcinogenic

before and after cisplatin administration. Maintain adequate hydration and urine output during next 24 hours.

• For patients with clinically significant third-space fluid, consider draining effusion before administering drug.

• To reduce toxicity, patient must take at least five daily doses of low-dose folic acid preparation or multivitamin with folic acid within 7 days before first pemetrexed dose.

• Reconstitute 500-mg vial with 20 ml preservative-free normal saline solution injection, yielding 25 mg/ml. Further dilute appropriate volume of reconstituted solution to 100 ml with preservative-free normal saline injection, and administer I.V. over 10 minutes.

• Drug is physically incompatible with diluents containing calcium.

• Patients with mild to moderate renal insufficiency should avoid taking NSAIDs for 5 days before, on day of, and for 2 days after pemetrexed administration.

• Monitor CBC and platelet count and periodic chemistry tests in all patients.

• Monitor for nadir and recovery before each dose and on days 8 and 15 of each treatment cycle. Do not start new cycle unless ANC is 1,500/mm³ or higher, platelet count is 100,000/mm³ or higher, and creatinine clearance is 45 ml/minute or higher.

---

pentostatin ⊠
Nipent

Indications and dosages
➡ Interferon alfa–refractory hairy cell leukemia
Adults: 4 mg/m² by I.V. bolus over 1 minute or diluted in larger volume and given over 20 to 30 minutes, every other week

Off-label uses (selected)

➡ Cutaneous T-cell lymphoma, including Sézary syndrome and mycosis fungoides
➡ Relapsed or refractory chronic lymphocytic leukemia

Special considerations
• Follow hazardous drug guidelines for preparation and administration.
• Withhold dose in patients with elevated serum creatinine level. In pa-

---

⊠ FDA black-box warning

tients with impaired renal function (creatinine clearance below 60 ml/minute), give drug only if potential benefit justifies potential risk.

• Withhold drug temporarily if absolute neutrophil count decreases from pretreatment baseline value above 500/mm^3 to below 200/mm^3 during therapy.

• Interrupt therapy temporarily if active infection occurs.

• Dose-limiting renal, hepatic, pulmonary, and CNS toxicities may occur.

• Using drug in combination with fludarabine phosphate in patients with refractory chronic lymphocytic leukemia is not recommended due to high risk of severe or fatal pulmonary toxicity.

• Before initiating therapy, obtain serum creatinine or creatinine clearance assay.

• Hydrate patient with 500 to 1,000 ml 5% dextrose in half-normal saline solution before drug is given. Administer additional 500 ml 5% dextrose solution or equivalent after drug is given.

• Inject 5 ml sterile water for injection into vial and mix thoroughly; yields 2 mg/ml solution.

• Give drug by I.V. bolus injection or dilute in larger volume (25 to 50 ml) with 5% dextrose injection or normal saline solution injection.

• Solution does not interact with PVC infusion containers or administration sets at concentrations of 0.18 to 0.33 mg/ml.

• Monitor CBC, blood chemistries, and serum creatinine level before each dose and at other appropriate times during therapy.

• Periodically monitor peripheral blood for hairy cells to evaluate response to treatment.

plicamycin (mithramycin) ⊠
Mithracin

Indications and dosages

➡ Testicular cancer in patients for whom successful treatment with surgery or radiation is impossible
Adults: Initially, 25 to 30 mcg/kg I.V. daily over 4 to 6 hours for 8 to 10 days, not to exceed 30 mcg/kg daily; may be repeated at monthly intervals if tumor mass remains unchanged. If significant testicular tumor regression occurs, give additional courses at monthly intervals until tu-

mor masses regress completely or new tumor masses show definite progression despite continued therapy.

➡ Reversal of hypercalcemia and hypercalciuria associated with advanced malignancy

Adults: 25 mcg/kg I.V. over 4 to 6 hours daily for 3 to 4 days; may be repeated weekly or on schedule of two or three doses weekly until adequate response occurs

Special considerations

• Follow hazardous drug guidelines for preparation and administration.
• Daily dosage is based on body weight. Use patient's ideal rather than actual weight.
• Drug is for I.V. use only.
• Due to possibility of severe reactions, drug should be given only to hospitalized patients.
• Before therapy begins, review data regarding drug use in treatment of testicular tumors and hypercalcemic or hypercalciuric conditions associated with various advanced cancers.
• Correct electrolyte imbalances, obtain renal function studies, and give antiemetic before therapy.
• To reconstitute, add 4.9 ml sterile water for injection to vial, to yield solution of 500 mcg/ml. Dilute calculated dose in 1 L 5% dextrose injection or normal saline solution injection.
• Give by slow I.V. infusion over 4 to 6 hours. Avoid rapid, direct I.V. injection.
• Extravasation may cause local irritation and cellulitis at injection site.
• Closely monitor hematologic function and observe patient for signs and symptoms of hemorrhagic syndrome.
• Continue to monitor renal and hepatic function and serum electrolytes closely during and after therapy.

---

porfimer sodium
Photofrin

Indications and dosages

➡ Palliation in completely obstructing esophageal cancer or in partially obstructing esophageal cancer in patients who cannot be satisfactorily treated with Nd:YAG laser therapy; reduction of obstruction and symp-

---

tom palliation in completely or partially obstructing endobronchial non-small-cell lung cancer; ablation of high-grade dysplasia in Barrett's esophagus in patients who do not undergo esophagectomy

Adults: Initially, 2 mg/kg as single, slow I.V. injection over 3 to 5 minutes; then, 40 to 50 hours later, laser light illumination at 630-nm wavelength; then residual tumor debridement followed by second laser light application 96 to 120 hours after initial drug injection. Patient may receive second photodynamic therapy (PDT) course no sooner than 30 days (90 days for dysplasia in Barrett's esophagus) after initial therapy. Up to three courses, each separated by at least 30 days (90 days for dysplasia in Barrett's esophagus), can be given.

➡ Microinvasive endobronchial non-small-cell lung cancer in patients for whom surgery and radiotherapy are not indicated

Adults: Initially, 2 mg/kg as single, slow I.V. injection over 3 to 5 minutes; then, 40 to 50 hours later, laser light illumination at 630-nm wavelength; then residual tumor debridement followed by second laser light application 96 to 120 hours after initial drug injection. Patient may receive second PDT course no sooner than 30 days after initial therapy. Up to three courses, each separated by at least 30 days, can be given.

OFF-LABEL USES (SELECTED)

➡ Transitional-cell carcinoma in situ of bladder

Special considerations

• Give drug as single, slow I.V. injection over 3 to 5 minutes.
• Reconstitute each vial with 31.8 ml 5% dextrose injection or normal saline solution injection.
• Take precautions to prevent extravasation at injection site.
• Before second laser light treatment, residual tumor should be debrided.
• PDT with porfimer is a two-stage process. Stage 1 is I.V. injection of drug. Stage 2 is illumination with 630-nm wavelength laser light.
• PDT is not suitable for patients with esophageal or gastric varices or esophageal ulcers larger than 1 cm in diameter.
• If PDT will precede radiotherapy, allow sufficient interval to ensure that inflammatory response from first treatment has subsided.
• Closely monitor patients with endobronchial lesions for respiratory distress between laser light therapy and mandatory debridement bronchoscopy.

⟩⟩ Potentially carcinogenic

procarbazine hydrochloride ⊠
Matulane

Indications and dosages

➡ Stage III or IV Hodgkin's lymphoma

Adults: As single agent, single or divided doses of 2 to 4 mg/kg P.O. daily for first week; then 4 to 6 mg/kg P.O. daily until maximum response occurs, WBC count decreases below 4,000/mm³, or platelet count drops below 100,000/mm³. When maximum response occurs, dosage may be maintained at 1 to 2 mg/kg/daily. In combination with nitrogen mustard, vincristine, procarbazine, and prednisone (MOPP regimen), procarbazine dosage is 100 mg/m² P.O. daily for 14 days.

Children: As single agent, 50 mg/m² P.O. daily for 7 days, followed by 100 mg/m² P.O. daily until desired response, leukopenia, or thrombocytopenia occurs. When response is maximal, 50 mg/m² P.O. daily as maintenance. As part of bleomycin, etoposide, doxorubicin, cyclophosphamide, vincristine, procarbazine, and prednisone (BEACOPP) regimen, procarbazine 100 mg/m² P.O. daily on days 1 to 7. Repeat cycle every 21 days.

Off-label uses (selected)

➡ Non-Hodgkin's lymphoma

➡ Progressive or recurrent nonresectable glioblastoma

➡ Small- and large-cell lung carcinomas, bronchogenic carcinoma, brain tumor, myeloma, melanoma, mycosis fungoides

Special considerations

⧫⧫ Follow hazardous drug guidelines for preparation and administration.

• If signs and symptoms of hematologic or other toxicity occur, discontinue drug until recovery. After toxic adverse effects subside, therapy may resume at 1 to 2 mg/kg P.O. daily.

• In children with Stage III or IV Hodgkin's lymphoma who have evidence of hematologic or other toxicity, discontinue drug until recovery.

• When used in combination with other anticancer drugs (as in MOPP regimen), dosage should be reduced appropriately.

• Dosages should be reduced in hepatic or renal failure.

• Therapy should be discontinued immediately if any of the following

⊠ FDA black-box warning

occur: CNS symptoms, such as paresthesia, neuropathies, or confusion; leukopenia (WBC count below 4,000/mm^3); thrombocytopenia (platelet count below 100,000/mm^3); hypersensitivity reaction; stomatitis (drug should be withdrawn at first small ulceration or persistent spot soreness in oral cavity); diarrhea; hemorrhage; or bleeding tendency.
• All dosages are based on actual weight.
• To decrease nausea, dose may be given at bedtime or in divided doses throughout day at beginning of therapy.
• In patients who have received radiation therapy or chemotherapeutic agents, wait at least 1 month before starting procarbazine.
• Monitor hematologic, renal, and hepatic function frequently.

raloxifene hydrochloride
Evista

Indications

OFF-LABEL USES (SELECTED)

➡ Reduction of incidence of estrogen-receptor-positive breast cancer

Special considerations
• Follow hazardous drug guidelines for preparation and administration.
• Drug may be given any time of day without regard to meals.
• Administer cautiously with other highly protein-bound drugs.
• Efficacy as chemopreventative measure for breast cancer in high-risk women has not been proven. Monitor these patients carefully.
• Monitor cholesterol, calcium, total protein, and platelet levels.

rituximab ⊠
Rituxan

Indications and dosages
➡ Relapsed or refractory low-grade or follicular, CD20+, B-cell non-Hodgkin's lymphoma
Adults: Initially, 375 mg/m^2 I.V. infusion once weekly for four or eight doses; in patients who subsequently develop progressive disease, 375 mg/m^2 I.V. infusion once weekly for four doses

⟫⟫ Potentially carcinogenic

OFF-LABEL USES (SELECTED)

➥ Chronic lymphocytic leukemia

Special considerations

• Acute renal failure requiring dialysis has been reported, in some cases leading to death from tumor lysis syndrome.

• Drug may be administered in outpatient settings.

• To administer, withdraw required amount and dilute to final concentration of 1 to 4 mg/ml into infusion bag containing normal saline solution or D_5W. Gently invert bag to mix solution.

• Do not mix or dilute with other drugs.

• Do not administer as I.V. push or bolus.

• During first infusion, administer I.V. at initial rate of 50 mg/hour.

• Stay alert for severe infusion reaction, which may be fatal.

• Unless hypersensitivity or infusion reaction occurs, increase infusion rate in 50-mg/hour increments every 30 minutes, to maximum of 400 mg/hour.

• Monitor CBC with differential and platelet counts at regular intervals during therapy.

• Continue to observe patient closely for signs of infusion reactions.

• Monitor for mucocutaneous reactions, arrhythmias, angina, and renal dysfunction.

• Monitor potassium and uric acid levels and observe for signs of tumor lysis syndrome, which can be fatal.

sodium phosphate P 32

Indications and dosages

➥ Chronic myeloid and chronic lymphocytic leukemia

Adults: 222 to 555 MBq (6 to 15 millicuries) I.V., usually given with hormone manipulation

➥ Palliative treatment of selected patients with multiple areas of skeletal metastasis

Adults: One regimen is 370 to 777 MBq (10 to 21 mCi) I.V. given over 3 to 4 weeks as 111 MBq (3 mCi) on day 1, followed by two doses of 74 MBq (2 mCi) every other day during first week, then two doses of 74 MBq (2 mCi) during second and third weeks, and then 37 MBq (1 mCi) twice weekly until total of 777 MBq (21 mCi) has been given.

Special considerations

- Follow hazardous drug guidelines for preparation and administration.
- Measure dosage by suitable radioactivity calibration immediately before use.
- Carefully ensure minimum radiation exposure to patient, consistent with proper patient management. Also ensure minimum radiation exposure to occupational workers.
- Visually inspect injection to avoid accidental I.V. administration of *chromic* phosphate P 32. Sodium phosphate P 32 is a clear, colorless solution; chromic phosphate P 32 is a green, cloudy liquid intended for intracavitary therapy.
- In women with childbearing potential, examinations using radiopharmaceuticals should be performed during first few (approximately 10) days after menses onset.
- Oral administration of high-specific-activity sodium phosphate P 32 in fasting state may equal I.V. administration.
- Monitor CBC and differential and bone marrow results frequently.

sorafenib
Nexavar

Indications and dosages
➡ Advanced renal-cell carcinoma
Adults: 400 mg P.O. twice daily given without food. Treatment should continue until no clinical benefit occurs or until unacceptable toxicity occurs.

OFF-LABEL USES (SELECTED)

➡ Recurrent epithelial ovarian cancer, advanced pancreatic cancer

Special considerations
- If severe or persistent hypertension occurs despite antihypertensive therapy or if cardiac ischemia occurs, consider temporary or permanent discontinuation of drug.
- Temporarily interrupt sorafenib therapy in patients undergoing major surgical procedures.
- If skin toxicity occurs, modify dosage.

- Monitor CBC with differential, platelets, hemoglobin, INR, and serum phosphate, amylase, lipase, and hepatic enzyme levels.
- Monitor blood pressure weekly during first 6 weeks of therapy and thereafter as needed.
- Monitor patient closely for hand-foot skin reactions.

streptozocin ⊠
Zanosar

Indications and dosages
➡ Metastatic islet-cell carcinoma of pancreas
Adults: 500 mg/m² I.V. daily for 5 consecutive days every 6 weeks until maximum benefit or treatment-limiting toxicity occurs (dosage increase not recommended). Weekly regimen is 1,000 mg/m² I.V. once weekly for 2 weeks; dosage may be increased in patients who did not achieve therapeutic response and did not experience significant toxicity during previous course, not to exceed single dose of 1,500 mg/m².

Special considerations
≫ Follow hazardous drug guidelines for preparation and administration.
- Dosages above 1,500 mg/m² may cause azotemia.
- Obtain baseline and serial urinalysis, BUN, serum creatinine and electrolyte levels, and creatinine clearance before therapy, at least weekly during therapy, and for 4 weeks afterward.
- Keep patient adequately hydrated to help reduce risk of nephrotoxicity.
- Extravasation may cause severe tissue lesions and necrosis.
- Administer by short I.V. infusion (over 10 to 15 minutes) or prolonged I.V. infusion (over 6 hours).
- Reconstitute with 9.5 ml dextrose injection or normal saline solution injection. When more dilute infusion solution is desirable, dilute further with same diluent.
- For patients with functional tumors, serial monitoring of fasting insulin level helps determine biochemical response to therapy.
- Drug commonly causes renal toxicity. Monitor renal function before and after each course. Adequate hydration may help reduce risk of nephrotoxicity to renal tubular epithelium.

strontium chloride Sr 89
Metastron

Indications and dosages
➥ Bone pain in patients with metastatic bone lesions
Adults: 148 MBq, 4 mCi, by slow I.V. injection over 1 or 2 minutes

Special considerations
• Follow hazardous drug guidelines for preparation and administration.
• Before therapy begins, bone metastases must be confirmed.
• Dose should be measured by suitable radioactivity calibration system immediately before administration.
• Base repeated administration on patient's response, current symptoms, and hematologic status.
• After administration, take special precautions in incontinent patients to minimize risk of radioactive contamination of clothing, bed linen, and other items.
• Monitor CBC with differential frequently.
• Closely monitor renal function.

tamoxifen citrate ⊠
Nolvadex

Indications and dosages
➥ Metastatic breast cancer in women and men, adjuvant treatment of breast cancer (treatment of axillary node–positive breast cancer in postmenopausal women after total or segmental mastectomy, axillary dissection, and breast irradiation; treatment of axillary node–negative breast cancer in women after total or segmental mastectomy, axillary dissection, and breast irradiation)
Adults: 20 to 40 mg P.O. daily; may be divided into two doses (morning and evening)
➥ To reduce risk of breast cancer in high-risk women; to reduce risk of invasive breast cancer in ductal carcinoma in situ (DCIS) after breast surgery and radiation
Adults: 20 mg P.O. daily for 5 years

⟫ Potentially carcinogenic

Off-label uses (selected)

➥ Hepatocellular carcinoma, other cancers with estrogen receptors

Special considerations

≫ Follow hazardous drug guidelines for preparation and administration.

• Serious and life-threatening events associated with drug in risk-reduction setting (women at high risk for cancer and women with DCIS) include uterine cancers, stroke, and pulmonary embolism. These events may be fatal.

• Monitor CBC and differential, liver function tests, and serum calcium and T_4 levels.

• Within a few weeks of starting drug, breast cancer patients with metastases may develop hypercalcemia.

• Ocular disturbances may occur.

• Drug has been associated with changes in liver enzyme levels and, in rare cases, more severe hepatic abnormalities.

• In sexually active women with childbearing potential, tamoxifen citrate therapy should be initiated during menstruation.

temozolomide
Temodar

Indications and dosages

➥ Newly diagnosed glioblastoma multiforme treated concomitantly with radiotherapy
Adults: Initially, 75 mg/m^2 P.O. daily for 42 days. Then, 4 weeks after completion of temozolomide and radiotherapy phase, 150 mg/m^2 P.O. daily for 5 days followed by 23 days without treatment (maintenance phase cycle 1). Then, at start of cycle 2, 200 mg/m^2 P.O. daily for first 5 days. Given for total of 6 cycles.
➥ Refractory anaplastic astrocytoma
Adults: 150 mg/m^2 P.O. daily for 5 days during 28-day cycle

Off-label uses (selected)

➥ Malignant glioma, metastatic melanoma

Special considerations

- Follow hazardous drug guidelines for preparation and administration.
- Dosage adjustment is based on nadir neutrophil and platelet counts.
- During treatment, obtain CBC on day 22 (21 days after first dose) or within 48 hours of that day, and weekly until absolute neutrophil count exceeds 1.5×10^9/L (1,500/mm³) and platelet count exceeds 100×10^9/L (100,000/mm³).
- To reduce nausea and vomiting, administer consistently on empty stomach.
- Monitor CBC and differential frequently.
- Higher incidence of *Pneumocystis carinii* pneumonia may occur when drug is given for prolonged period.

teniposide ⊠
Vumon

Indications and dosages

➡ Refractory childhood acute lymphoblastic leukemia

Children: Teniposide 165 mg/m² I.V. infusion in combination with cytarabine 300 mg/m² I.V. infusion twice weekly for eight or nine doses; or in combination with vincristine and prednisone, teniposide 250 mg/m² I.V. infusion with vincristine 1.5 mg/m² I.V. infusion weekly for 4 to 8 weeks and prednisone 40 mg/m² P.O. daily for 28 days

OFF-LABEL USES (SELECTED)

➡ Refractory non-Hodgkin's lymphoma
➡ Neuroblastoma
➡ Small-cell lung cancer

Special considerations

》》 Follow hazardous drug guidelines for preparation and administration.
- Patients with both Down syndrome and leukemia may be especially sensitive to drug.
- Patients receiving two or more bone marrow–depressant therapies (including radiation) concurrently or consecutively may require dosage reductions.
- Evaluate CBC and differential, platelet count, hemoglobin, and kidney

》》 Potentially carcinogenic

and liver function tests carefully before therapy starts.
• If undiluted injection concentrate comes in contact with plastic equipment or devices used to prepare solutions for infusion, plastic may soften or crack and product leakage may occur.
• Dilute with 5% dextrose injection or normal saline solution injection for final concentration of 0.1 mg/ml, 0.2 mg/ml, 0.4 mg/ml, or 1 mg/ml. Give solutions prepared at final concentration of 1 mg/ml within 4 hours to reduce risk of precipitation.
• Precipitation may occur during 24-hour infusions diluted to concentrations of 0.1 to 0.2 mg/ml, causing occlusion of central venous access catheter. To prevent these problems, flush administration apparatus thoroughly with 5% dextrose injection or normal saline solution injection before and after drug administration.
• Give drug only by slow I.V. infusion lasting at least 30 to 60 minutes.
• With first dose, hypersensitivity reaction may occur. Reaction may be life-threatening if not treated promptly.
• Dose-limiting bone marrow depression is most significant toxicity.
• At start of therapy and before each subsequent dose, monitor hemoglobin, WBC count and differential, and platelet count.
• Monitor plasma albumin level, platelet count, hemoglobin, and kidney and liver function tests carefully throughout therapy.
• Observe for acute CNS depression and hypotension in patients receiving high doses who have been pretreated with antiemetics.
• Observe patient; be prepared for possible hypersensitivity reaction throughout therapy.

---

testolactone
Teslac

Indications and dosages
➥ Adjunctive therapy in palliative treatment of advanced or disseminated breast cancer in postmenopausal women when hormonal therapy is indicated
Adults: 250 mg P.O. four times daily

Special considerations
• Follow hazardous drug guidelines for preparation and administration.
• Monitor patient routinely for hypercalcemia.

☒ FDA black-box warning

• Discontinue therapy for at least 3 months to evaluate response unless active disease progression occurs.

thalidomide ⊠
Thalomid

Indications

OFF-LABEL USES (SELECTED)

➥ Advanced refractory multiple myeloma
➥ Prostate cancer
➥ Clinical manifestations of Kaposi's sarcoma or primary brain malignancies
➥ Recurrent glioblastoma multiforme of CNS

Special considerations

• Follow hazardous drug guidelines for preparation and administration.
• If taken during pregnancy, drug can cause severe birth defects or fetal death. It should never be used by women who are pregnant or could become pregnant during therapy.
• To reduce chance of fetal exposure, drug is approved only under special restricted distribution program approved by FDA (System for Thalidomide Education and Prescribing Safety, or STEPS).
• Reliable contraception is required even if patient has a history of infertility, unless she has had a hysterectomy or has been postmenopausal for at least 24 months.
• In women with childbearing potential, use hinges on initial and continued confirmed negative pregnancy tests.
• Monitor WBC with differential frequently.
• Observe closely for hypersensitivity reactions.

thioguanine ⊠
Tabloid

Indications and dosages

➥ Acute nonlymphocytic leukemia
Adults and children age 3 and older: 2 mg/kg P.O. daily; if no clinical

≫ Potentially carcinogenic

improvement occurs after 4 weeks, increase dosage slowly to 3 mg/kg daily.

➥ Chronic myelogenous leukemia

Special considerations

• Follow hazardous drug guidelines for preparation and administration.

• Drug should be discontinued temporarily at first sign of abnormally steep fall in any formed blood element.

• Decision to increase, decrease, continue, or discontinue a given dosage must be based not only on absolute hematologic values but also on how fast these values are changing.

• Thioguanine is a potent drug and should not be used unless diagnosis of acute nonlymphocytic leukemia has been adequately established and responsible physician knows how to assess patient's response to chemotherapy.

• Monitor hemoglobin, hematocrit, WBC and differential counts, and quantitative platelet counts frequently during therapy.

thiotepa

Indications and dosages

➥ Adenocarcinoma of breast or ovary, Hodgkin's lymphoma, other lymphomas
Adults: 0.3 to 0.4 mg/kg by rapid I.V. administration at 1- to 4-week intervals
➥ Intracavitary effusion secondary to diffuse or localized neoplastic disease
Adults: 0.6 to 0.8 mg/kg intracavitary (usually a one-time infusion)
➥ Superficial papillary urinary bladder carcinoma
Adults: 60 mg in 60 ml sodium chloride injection (normal saline solution) instilled in bladder by catheter and retained for 2 hours, once weekly for 4 weeks; repeated monthly if necessary

➥ Autologous bone marrow transplantation
➥ Carcinomatous meningitis

⊠ FDA black-box warning

Special considerations

▶▶ Follow hazardous drug guidelines for preparation and administration.

• Discontinue therapy if WBC count falls to 3,000/mm³ or lower or platelet count falls to 150,000/mm³.

• For I.V. use, reconstitute each 15 mg with 1.5 ml sterile water for injection to yield 10 mg/ml. Dilute further with normal saline solution before use.

• In papillary bladder carcinoma, dehydrate patient for 8 to 12 hours before treatment.

• Administer at a rate of 60 mg (or fraction thereof) by I.V. injection over 1 minute.

• Obtain weekly WBC with differential and platelet counts during therapy and for at least 3 weeks afterward.

• Carefully monitor patients with hepatic or renal impairment.

topotecan hydrochloride ☒
Hycamtin

Indications and dosages

➡ Metastatic ovarian carcinoma and small-cell lung cancer after chemotherapy failure

Adults: 1.5 mg/m² I.V. infusion given over 30 minutes for 5 consecutive days, starting on day 1 of 21-day course and given for at least four courses unless tumor progresses; reduced by 0.25 mg/m² for subsequent courses if severe neutropenia occurs or if platelet count falls below 25,000/mm³

Off-label uses (selected)

➡ Non-small-cell lung cancer (evidence rating IIIA)
➡ Myelodysplastic syndrome (evidence rating II/IIID)
➡ Chronic myelomonocytic leukemia (evidence rating IIID)

Special considerations

• Follow hazardous drug guidelines for preparation and administration.
• Drug is not recommended as first-line therapy for non-small-cell lung cancer.

▶▶ Potentially carcinogenic

- Dosage adjustment to 0.75 mg/m² is recommended for patients with moderate renal impairment.
- Patients should not receive subsequent courses until neutrophil count recovers to above 1,000/mm³, platelet count to above 100,000/mm³, and hemoglobin to or above 9 g/dl.
- Before first course, patients must have baseline neutrophil count above 1,500/mm³ and platelet count above 100,000/mm³.
- Reconstitute each 4-mg vial with 4 ml sterile water for injection. Then dilute appropriate volume of reconstituted solution in normal saline solution for I.V. infusion or 5% dextrose for I.V. infusion.
- Extravasation has been associated with mild erythema and bruising.
- Neutropenia is dose-limiting toxicity and is not cumulative over time. Monitor CBC with differential frequently.
- Monitor renal and hepatic function, especially in elderly patients.

toremifene citrate
Fareston

Indications and dosages
➥ Metastatic breast cancer in postmenopausal women with estrogen-receptor positive or unknown tumors
Adults: 60 mg P.O. daily

Special considerations
- Follow hazardous drug guidelines for preparation and administration.
- Because of drug's extensive hepatic transformation, dosage adjustments may be needed in patients with hepatic impairment.
- Monitor CBC, calcium level, and liver function tests periodically.
- Tumor flare may occur in breast cancer patients with bone metastases during first weeks of therapy.

tositumomab and iodine ¹³¹I tositumomab ☒
Bexxar Dosimetric, Bexxar ¹³¹I Dosimetric, Bexxar ¹³¹I Therapeutic, Bexxar Therapeutic

Indications and dosages
➥ CD20+ follicular non-Hodgkin's lymphoma, with and without

transformation, when disease is refractory to rituximab and has relapsed after chemotherapy

Adults: Bexxar therapeutic regimen has four components in two steps—dosimetric step, followed 7 to 14 days later by therapeutic step. *Dosimetric step:* (1) Tositumomab 450 mg I.V. in 50 ml normal saline solution over 60 minutes. (2) Iodine ^{131}I tositumomab (containing 5.0 mCi ^{131}I and 35 mg tositumomab) I.V. in 30 ml normal saline solution over 20 minutes.

Therapeutic step: (Do not administer this step if biodistribution is altered. For assessment information regarding biodistribution, see manufacturer's prescribing information.)

(1) Tositumomab 450 mg I.V. in 50 ml normal saline solution over 60 minutes. (2) ^{131}I tositumomab: See manufacturer's prescribing information for calculating iodine ^{131}I activity.

Special considerations

• Follow hazardous drug guidelines for preparation and administration.
Note: See manufacturer's prescribing information for guidelines on qualifications to administer, radiation precautions, preparation, and dose calibrations.

• *Patients with infusion reactions:* Reduce infusion rate 50% for mild to moderate infusional toxicity; interrupt infusion for severe infusional toxicity.

• *Patients with platelet count of 150,000/mm^3 or higher:* Recommended dosage is ^{131}I activity calculated to deliver 75 cGy total body irradiation and 35 mg tositumomab, given I.V. over 20 minutes.

• *Patients with NCI Grade 1 thrombocytopenia (platelet count above 100,000/mm^3 but below 150,000/mm^3):* Recommended dosage is ^{131}I activity calculated to deliver 65 cGy total body irradiation and 35 mg tositumomab, given I.V. over 20 minutes.

• Most patients who receive Bexxar therapeutic regimen experienced severe thrombocytopenia and neutropenia.

• Bexxar therapeutic regimen can cause fetal harm when given to pregnant patients.

• Obtain CBC with differential and platelet count before administering Bexxar therapeutic regimen.

• Administer Bexxar therapeutic regimen through I.V. tubing set with inline 0.22-micron filter.

◆◆ Potentially carcinogenic

• Use same I.V. tubing set and filter during entire dosimetric or therapeutic step. Filter change could cause drug loss.

• Patients should not receive dosimetric dose unless they have received the following medications: Thyroid-protective agents, acetaminophen, and diphenhydramine.

• Safety of Bexxar therapeutic regimen has been established only in patients receiving thyroid-blocking agents and premedication to reduce or prevent infusion reactions.

• Safety of Bexxar therapeutic regimen has not been established in patients with more than 25% lymphoma marrow involvement, platelet count below 100,000/mm³, or neutrophil count below 1,500/mm³.

• Continue weekly monitoring of CBC with differential for at least 10 weeks after Bexxar therapeutic regimen.

• Impaired renal function may decrease ^{131}I excretion rate and increase patient exposure to radioactive component.

trastuzumab ⊠
Herceptin

Indications and dosages

➡ Metastatic breast cancer in patients with tumors that overexpress human epidermal growth factor receptor 2 protein (HER2) and who have received one or more chemotherapy regimens; in combination with paclitaxel for treatment of patients with metastatic breast cancer whose tumors overexpress HER2 and who have not received chemotherapy for metastatic disease

Adults: As single agent and in combination therapy, trastuzumab 4 mg/kg I.V. infusion over 90 minutes, followed by 2 mg/kg I.V. infusion over 30 minutes once weekly as maintenance; in combination therapy, paclitaxel dosage is 175 mg/m² I.V. over 3 hours every 21 days for at least six cycles.

OFF-LABEL USES (SELECTED)

➡ Metastatic breast cancer in patients with tumors that overexpress HER2 and who have received one or more chemotherapy regimens
➡ Adjuvant treatment in patients with surgically removed HER2-positive breast cancer

Special considerations

• Drug can cause ventricular dysfunction and heart failure and severe hypersensitivity reactions.
• Do not give by I.V. push or bolus.
• Do not mix with other drugs or with dextrose solutions.
• Reconstitute each vial with 20 ml bacteriostatic water for injection, 1.1% benzyl alcohol preserved, as supplied, to yield multidose solution containing 21 mg/ml.
• Immediately after reconstitution, label vial in the area marked "Do not use after:" with date that is 28 days from reconstitution date.
• Observe patient for fever, chills, and other infusion-associated reactions. If severe reaction occurs, interrupt infusion and provide supportive therapy.
• Severe infusion reaction typically occurs with initial infusion and generally arises during or immediately after infusion.

tretinoin, all-*trans* retinoic acid (ATRA) ⊠
Vesanoid

Indications and dosages

➡ Acute promyelocytic leukemia (APL) classified M3 by French-American-British system, characterized by presence of t(15:17) translocation and/or PML/RARα gene in patients who are refractory to or have relapsed from anthracycline chemotherapy or for whom anthracycline chemotherapy is contraindicated
Adults and children age 1 and older: 45 mg/m^2 P.O. daily in two evenly divided doses, discontinued after either 90 days or 30 days after complete remission occurs, whichever comes first

Special considerations

• Follow hazardous drug guidelines for preparation and administration.
• Dosage reduction should be considered for children with serious or intolerable toxicity.
• Drug is used only to induce remission.
• Monitor patient for serious adverse reactions, including retinoic acid–APL syndrome and leukocytosis.
• Pseudotumor cerebri may occur, particularly in children.

⟫ Potentially carcinogenic

triptorelin pamoate
Trelstar Depot, Trelstar LA

Indications and dosages
➥ Palliative treatment of advanced prostate cancer
Adults: 3.75 mg (depot) I.M. every 4 weeks as single injection; or 11.25 mg (long-acting) I.M. every 12 weeks as single injection

Special considerations
• Follow hazardous drug guidelines for preparation and administration.
• Monitor serum levels of testosterone and prostate-specific antigen immediately before and during dosing to determine response to therapy.
• Reconstitute microgranules with sterile water. Do not use other diluents.
• Discard suspension if it is not used immediately after reconstitution.
• Rotate I.M. injection sites.
• Transient serum testosterone increase may be associated with temporary worsening of prostate cancer symptoms during first weeks of treatment.
• Drug has caused spinal cord compression, which may contribute to paralysis with or without fatal complications.
• Patients with renal or hepatic impairment may show two- to fourfold higher exposure than healthy young males. Monitor kidney and liver function tests.

valrubicin
Valstar

Indications and dosages
➥ Bacillus Calmette-Guérin–refractory urinary bladder cancer in patients for whom immediate cystectomy is unacceptable
Adults: 800 mg intravesically every week for 6 weeks, starting 14 or more days after fulguration or transurethral resection

Special considerations
• Follow hazardous drug guidelines for preparation and administration.

⊠ FDA black-box warning

• For each instillation, dilute 20 ml of drug with 55 ml normal saline solution injection, yielding 75 ml of diluted solution.

• For intravesical instillation, urethral catheter is inserted into bladder under aseptic conditions. Bladder is drained, and diluted 75-ml valrubicin solution is instilled slowly by gravity flow over several minutes. Catheter is then withdrawn. Patient should retain drug for 2 hours.

• Ensure that patient maintains adequate hydration after treatment.

• Do not clamp catheter in patients with severe irritable bladder symptoms, including spasms.

• Evaluate patient for bladder rupture.

vinblastine sulfate ⊠

Indications and dosages

➡ Palliative treatment of advanced testicular cancer, Hodgkin's disease (Stages III and IV, Ann Arbor modification of Rye staging system), lymphocytic lymphoma, histiocytic lymphoma, mycosis fungoides, histiocytosis, Kaposi's sarcoma, choriocarcinoma resistant to other chemotherapeutic agents, breast carcinoma unresponsive to appropriate endocrine surgery and hormonal therapy

Adults: 0.1 mg/kg or 3.7 mg/m^2 I.V. weekly or every 2 weeks, not to exceed 0.5 mg/kg or 18.5 mg/m^2 weekly

Children: Initially 2.5 mg/m^2 I.V., followed by 3.75 mg/m^2, 5 mg/m^2, 6.25 mg/m^2, and then 7.5 mg/m^2 I.V. at 7-day intervals

Off-label uses (selected)

➡ Bladder, cervical, and head and neck cancer

➡ Melanoma

➡ Non-small-cell lung cancer

➡ Germ cell tumors

Special considerations

• Follow hazardous drug guidelines for preparation and administration.

• Hematologic intolerance should guide dosage.

• Dosage reduction of 50% is recommended for patients with direct serum bilirubin level above 3 mg/dl.

• Drug is for I.V. use only and is fatal if given intrathecally. I.V. needle or catheter must be properly positioned before drug is injected.

⊠ Potentially carcinogenic

• With inadvertent intrathecal administration, immediate neurosurgical intervention is needed to prevent ascending paralysis leading to death.

• Syringe containing specific dose must be labeled, using auxiliary sticker provided, "Fatal if given intrathecally. For I.V. use only."

• Reconstitute powder with 10 ml normal saline solution to concentration of 1 mg/ml. Inject I.V. dose into tubing of running I.V. line or by direct injection over 1 minute.

• Except in off-label uses, give no more often than once every 7 days.

• To initiate therapy in adults, administer single I.V. dose of 3.7 mg/m² (except in off-label uses). Thereafter, obtain WBC count to determine patient's sensitivity to drug.

• Watch for infection in patients with WBC counts below 2,000/mm³.

• In patients with malignant-cell infiltration of bone marrow, WBC and platelet counts may fall precipitously after moderate doses. Further drug use in such patients is inadvisable.

• If acute respiratory problems occur, do not readminister drug.

---

vincristine sulfate ⊠
Oncovin, Vincasar PFS

Indications and dosages

➡ Hodgkin's disease, non-Hodgkin's lymphoma, acute leukemia, nephroblastoma, rhabdomyosarcoma
Adults: 0.03 to 1.4 mg/m² I.V. weekly; maximum dosage is 2 mg.
Children weighing more than 10 kg (22 lb): 1.5 to 2 mg/m² I.V. weekly (varies with protocol)
Children weighing 10 kg (22 lb) or less: 0.05 mg/kg I.V. weekly (varies with protocol)

OFF-LABEL USES (SELECTED)

➡ AIDS-related Kaposi's sarcoma, intracranial tumor, hepatic carcinoma, small-cell lung carcinoma, testicular cancer, ovarian cancer, malignant pheochromocytoma

Special considerations

⯈⯈ Follow hazardous drug guidelines for preparation and administration.

⊠ FDA black-box warning

- Dosage reduction of 50% is recommended for patients with direct serum bilirubin concentrations above 3 mg/dl.
- Dosage limitation depends on patient response and protocol used.
- If intrathecal administration occurs, treatment includes immediate removal of CSF and flushing with lactated Ringer's or other solution. Treatment must begin immediately after intrathecal injection.
- Syringe containing specific dose must be labeled, using auxiliary sticker provided, "Fatal if given intrathecally. For I.V. use only."
- Drug is for I.V. use only. Administer dose through intact, free-flowing I.V. needle or catheter within 1 minute.
- Ensure that I.V. needle or catheter is properly positioned before drug injection, to prevent extravasation.
- Monitor CBC before each dose.
- Monitor serum uric acid level during first 3 to 4 weeks of therapy.
- If acute respiratory problems occur, do not readminister drug.

vinorelbine tartrate ⊠
Navelbine

Indications and dosages
➥ Unresectable, advanced (stage IV) non-small-cell lung cancer
Adults: As single agent, 30 mg/m² I.V. given over 6 to 10 minutes every week. Vinorelbine 30 mg/m² I.V. may be given weekly in combination with cisplatin on days 1 and 29, then every 6 weeks at a dosage of 120 mg/m²; or vinorelbine 25 mg/m² I.V. may be given weekly in combination with cisplatin administered every 4 weeks.
➥ Unresectable, advanced (stage III) non-small-cell lung cancer stage
Adults: As combination therapy, vinorelbine 30 mg/m² I.V. may be given weekly in combination with cisplatin on days 1 and 29, then every 6 weeks at a dosage of 120 mg/m²; or vinorelbine 25 mg/m² I.V. weekly in combination with cisplatin given every 4 weeks.

OFF-LABEL USES (SELECTED)
➥ Metastatic breast cancer, recurrent ovarian cancer, cervical cancer

Special considerations
- Follow hazardous drug guidelines for preparation and administration.

⟫ Potentially carcinogenic

- Dosage should be adjusted according to hematologic toxicity or hepatic insufficiency (hyperbilirubinemia).
- Reduce dosage to 50% of starting dosage if granulocyte count is 1,000 to 1,499/mm³ on day of treatment. If patient experiences fever or sepsis on initial therapy or if two consecutive doses were withheld because of granulocytopenia, subsequent doses should be 75% of starting dosage for absolute neutrophil count (ANC) of 1,500/mm³ or more. If ANC is 1,000 to 1,499/mm³, dosage should be 37.5% of starting dosage.
- In patients with total bilirubin level of 2.1 to 3 mg/dl, use 50% of starting dosage. For total bilirubin level above 3 mg/dl, use 25% of starting dosage.
- If Grade 2 or higher neurotoxicity develops, discontinue drug.
- Product is for I.V. use only. Intrathecal administration may result in death. Syringes containing drug should be labeled, "Warning—for I.V. use only. Fatal if given intrathecally."
- Severe granulocytopenia may occur.
- Drug administration may result in extravasation, causing severe local tissue necrosis, thrombophlebitis, or both.
- For I.V. injection, dilute each 10 mg (1 ml) in syringe with at least 2 to 5 ml normal saline for injection or D_5W for desired concentration of 1.5 to 3 mg/ml. Administer diluted drug over 6 to 10 minutes into side port of free-flowing I.V. line closest to I.V. bag; then flush with at least 75 to 125 ml of recommended solution.
- For intermittent I.V. infusion, dilute each 10 mg (1 ml) with 4 to 19 ml normal saline for injection, D_5W, half-normal saline solution, D_5W in half-normal saline solution, Ringer's solution, or lactated Ringer's solution for desired concentration of 0.5 to 2 mg/ml. Administer diluted drug over 6 to 20 minutes into side port of free-flowing I.V. line, or give directly into large central vein and then flush with at least 75 to 125 ml of recommended solution.
- Monitor patient for myelosuppression during and after therapy.
- Acute dyspnea and severe bronchospasm may occur.
- Potentially fatal interstitial pulmonary changes and adult respiratory distress syndrome may occur with single-agent therapy.
- Drug may cause severe constipation, paralytic ileus, intestinal obstruction, necrosis, or perforation.
- If patient has history of or preexisting neuropathy, monitor closely for new or worsening signs and symptoms of neuropathy during therapy.
- "Radiation recall" may occur if drug is given after radiation therapy.

☒ FDA black-box warning

Chemotherapy regimens and supportive therapy

Generally, combination chemotherapy is more effective than single-agent chemotherapy. Each drug used in a combination regimen should be effective alone against the specific cancer and should potentiate the effects of other drugs in the combination.

For most cancers, optimum treatment schedules have not been established. However, sequence and timing of drug administration are crucial because the goal is to affect the largest numbers of cells during their susceptible phase. Use of supportive therapies also influences the success of therapy by allowing patients to better tolerate toxic effects of chemotherapeutic agents and experience improved quality of life.

Selected regimens

Hundreds of combination chemotherapy regimens exist. The regimens listed here are among the most commonly used. The selection is not meant to be all-inclusive or to direct a practitioner's specific choice of therapy; nor do the authors or publisher endorse or recommend any specific regimen. (Regimens for children are not included because, for most children, treatment is based on a national group protocol.)

Determining which regimen is best for a particular patient is based on professional judgment, experience, and the patient's diagnosis and clinical status; one must carefully weigh the regimen's anticipated benefits against potential risks.

Organization

This section is arranged alphabetically by neoplastic disease. Within each disease entry, chemotherapy regimens are listed alphabetically by drug names. Shortened references follow each regimen; some pertain to the original study, others to follow-up investigations or trials. (For the complete references, visit www.oncologydrugguide.com.)

For each regimen, you will find a list of complications that the regimen is likely to cause—for example, nausea and vomiting, myelosuppression, dehydration, diarrhea, anemia, or neutropenia. For more information on treatment guidelines for supportive therapies, see the appendices.

Acute myeloid leukemia

AIDA (all-*trans* retinoic acid, idarubicin) for promyelocytic leukemia

All-trans retinoic acid (ATRA) 45 mg/m² P.O. daily until complete remission or maximum of 90 days and *idarubicin* 12 mg/m² I.V. on days 2, 4, 6, and 8

Followed by three monthly consolidation cycles—
First cycle: *idarubicin* 5 mg/m² I.V. daily on days 1 through 4
Second cycle: mitoxantrone 10 mg/m² I.V. daily on days 1 through 5
Third cycle: *idarubicin* 12 mg/m² I.V. on day 1 only

Follow consolidation cycles with maintenance therapy until polymerase chain reaction is negative—

ATRA 45 mg/m² P.O. for 15 days every 3 months with or without methotrexate 15 mg/m² P.O. weekly and 6-mercaptopurine (6-MP) 90 mg/m² P.O. daily

Continue maintenance therapy for 2 years.

Reference: Sanz MA, et al. *Blood.* 1999;94:3015-3021; Avvisati G, et al. *Blood.* 1996;88:1390-1398.

Supportive therapy

Patients are at moderate to high risk for nausea and vomiting and neutropenia. Supportive and/or prophylactic therapies are recommended.

Cytarabine, daunorubicin (7+3)

Cytarabine 100 mg/m² I.V. daily for 7 days
Daunorubicin 45 mg/m² I.V. daily on days 1 through 3
   After 14 days, if more than 5% of remaining nucleated cells are leukemic, give:
Cytarabine 100 mg/m² I.V. daily for 5 days
Daunorubicin 45 mg/m² I.V. daily on days 1 and 2

Reference: Volger WR. *J Clin Oncol.* 1992;10:1103-1111; Mayer RJ. *N Engl J Med.* 1994;331:896-903.

Supportive therapy

Patients are at moderate to high risk for nausea and vomiting, neutropenia, and diarrhea. Supportive and/or prophylactic therapies are recommended.

See appendices for supportive therapies.

Gemtuzumab

Gemtuzumab 6 to 9 mg/m^2 I.V. over 2 hours on days 1 and 15. Third dose may be given if bone marrow polymerase chain reaction is negative.

Reference: Lo Coco F, et al. *Blood.* 2004;104:1995-1999; Larson RA, et al. *Leukemia.* 2002;16:1627-1636.

Supportive therapy

Patients are at moderate to high risk for nausea and vomiting, neutropenia, and infusion reactions. Supportive and/or prophylactic therapies are recommended.

HDAC, HiDAC (high-dose cytarabine)

Cytarabine 3 g/m^2 I.V. over 3 hours every 12 hours on days 1, 3, and 5
Give for four cycles.
Reference: Cassileth PA, et al. *N Engl J Med.* 1998;339:1649-1656.

Supportive therapy

Patients are at moderate to high risk for nausea and vomiting, neutropenia, diarrhea, and conjunctivitis. Supportive and/or prophylactic therapies are recommended.

Bladder cancer

Cisplatin, docetaxel

Cisplatin 75 mg/m^2 I.V. on day 1
Docetaxel 75 mg/m^2 I.V. on day 1
Repeat cycle every 21 days.
Reference: Dimopoulos MA, et al. *Ann Oncol.* 1999;10:1385-1388; Sengelov L, et al. *J Clin Oncol.* 1998;3392-3397.

Supportive therapy

Patients are at moderate to high risk for nausea and vomiting, anemia, neutropenia, hypersensitivity reactions, and cisplatin-induced nephrotoxicity. Supportive and/or prophylactic therapies are recommended.

CMV (cisplatin, methotrexate, vinblastine)

Methotrexate 30 to 40 mg/m^2 I.V. on days 1 and 8
Vinblastine 4 mg/m^2 I.V. on days 1 and 8
Cisplatin 100 mg/m^2 I.V. over 4 hours on day 2
Repeat cycle every 21 days.

Reference: Harker WG, et al. *J Clin Oncol.* 1985;3:1463-1470; Wie CH, et al. *J Urol.* 1996;155:118-125.

Supportive therapy

Patients are at moderate to high risk for nausea and vomiting, anemia, neutropenia, diarrhea, and cisplatin-induced nephrotoxicity. Supportive and/or prophylactic therapies are recommended.

Gemcitabine

Gemcitabine 1,200 mg/m^2 I.V on, days 1, 8, and 15
Repeat every 28 days for maximum of six cycles.

Reference: von der Maase H. *Crit Rev Oncol Hematol.* 2000;34(3):175-183.

Supportive therapy

Patients are at moderate to high risk for nausea and vomiting and anemia. Supportive and/or prophylactic therapies are recommended.

Gemcitabine, cisplatin

Gemcitabine 1,000 mg/m^2 I.V. on days 1, 8, and 15
Cisplatin 70 mg/m^2 I.V. on day 2
Repeat cycle every 28 days for maximum of six cycles.

Reference: von der Masse H, et al. *J Clin Oncol.* 2000;17:3068-3077.

Supportive therapy

Patients are at moderate to high risk for nausea and vomiting, anemia, neutropenia, and cisplatin-induced nephrotoxicity. Supportive and/or prophylactic therapies are recommended.

ITP (ifosfamide, paclitaxel [Taxol], cisplatin [Platinol-AQ])

Ifosfamide 1,500 mg/m^2 I.V. on days 1 through 3 with mesna 300 mg/m^2 I.V. for three doses (30 minutes before start of ifosfamide, 4 hours later, and 8 hours later) on days 1 through 3

Paclitaxel 200 mg/m^2 I.V. over 3 hours on day 1

Cisplatin 70 mg/m^2 on day 1

Repeat cycle every 28 days.

Reference: Bajorin DF. *Cancer.* 2000;88:1671-1678.

Supportive therapy

Patients are at moderate to high risk for nausea and vomiting, anemia, neutropenia, hypersensitivity reactions, and cisplatin-induced nephrotoxicity. Supportive and/or prophylactic therapies are recommended.

MVAC (methotrexate, vinblastine, doxorubicin [Adriamycin], cisplatin)

Methotrexate 30 mg/m^2 I.V. on days 1, 15, and 22

Vinblastine 3 mg/m^2 I.V. on days 2, 15, and 22

Doxorubicin 30 mg/m^2 I.V. on day 2

Cisplatin 70 mg/m^2 I.V. on day 2

Repeat cycle every 28 days.

Reference: von der Masse H, et al. *J Clin Oncol.* 2000;17:3068-3077.

Supportive therapy

Patients are at moderate to high risk for nausea and vomiting, neutropenia, and cisplatin-induced nephrotoxicity. Supportive and/or prophylactic therapies are recommended.

Paclitaxel

Paclitaxel 250 mg/m^2 I.V. over 24 hours on day 1

Repeat every 21 days.

Reference: Roth BJ, et al. *J Clin Oncol.* 1994;12:2264-2270.

Supportive therapy

Patients are at moderate to high risk for nausea and vomiting, anemia, neutropenia, and hypersensitivity reactions. Supportive and/or prophylactic therapies are recommended.

PC (paclitaxel, carboplatin)

Paclitaxel 225 mg/m^2 I.V. over 3 hours on day 1
Carboplatin to AUC of 6 mg/ml/minute I.V. on day 1, given 15 minutes after paclitaxel
Repeat cycle every 21 days.

Reference: Dreicer R. *Cancer.* 2004;100:1639-1645.

Supportive therapy

Patients are at moderate to high risk for nausea and vomiting, neutropenia, hypersensitivity reactions, and cisplatin-induced nephrotoxicity. Supportive and/or prophylactic therapies are recommended.

Bone sarcoma

CAV (cyclophosphamide, doxorubicin [Adriamycin], vincristine) alternating with IE (ifosfamide, etoposide)

CAV

Cyclophosphamide 1,200 mg/m^2 I.V. and mesna 240 mg/m^2 I.V. on day 1; repeat mesna every 3 hours for three to four doses
Doxorubicin 75 mg/m^2 I.V. on day 1 (after 375 mg/m^2 cumulative dose of doxorubicin, substitute dactinomycin 1.25 mg/m^2 I.V.)
Vincristine 2 mg I.V. on day 1

IE

Ifosfamide 1,800 mg/m^2 I.V. with mesna 360 mg/m^2 I.V. for three doses (given initially with ifosfamide, then 4 hours later, and 8 hours later) on days 1 through 5
Etoposide 100 mg/m^2 I.V. on days 1 through 5
Alternate CAV with IE regimens every 21 days for total of 17 cycles.

Reference: Holcombe E, et al. *N Engl J Med.* 2003;348:694-671.

Supportive therapy

Patients are at moderate to high risk for nausea and vomiting and neutropenia. Supportive and/or prophylactic therapies are recommended.

Breast cancer

AC (doxorubicin [Adriamycin], cyclophosphamide)

Doxorubicin 60 mg/m^2 I.V. on day 1
Cyclophosphamide 600 mg/m^2 I.V. on day 1
Repeat cycle every 21 days.

Reference: Fisher B, et al. *J Clin Oncol.* 1990;8:2150-2156; Fisher B, et al. *J Clin Oncol.* 1997;15:1858-1869.

Supportive therapy

Patients are at moderate to high risk for nausea and vomiting and neutropenia. Supportive and/or prophylactic therapies are recommended.

Bevacizumab, paclitaxel

Bevacizumab 10 mg/kg I.V. over 90 minutes on days 1 and 15; if tolerated, may decrease rate of infusion to 30 to 60 minutes
Paclitaxel 90 mg/m^2 I.V. on days 1, 8, and 15
Repeat cycle every 28 days.

Reference: Sledge GW. *Breast Cancer Update* [Online]. 2005; Shulman LN, et al. *Medscape.* 2005; Miller KD, et al. Presentation at ASCO Meeting; 2005.

Supportive therapy

Patients are at moderate to high risk for nausea and vomiting and hypersensitivity reactions. Supportive and/or prophylactic therapies are recommended.

Capecitabine

Capecitabine 1,250 mg/m^2 P.O. twice daily on days 1 through 14
Repeat every 21 days.

Reference: Fumoleau P, et al. *Eur J Cancer.* 2004;40:536-542.

Supportive therapy

Patients are at moderate to high risk for nausea and vomiting, anemia, neutropenia, and diarrhea. Supportive and/or prophylactic therapies are recommended.

CMF (cyclophosphamide, methotrexate, 5-fluorouracil)

Patients younger than age 60:

Cyclophosphamide 100 mg/m^2 P.O. on days 1 through 14

Methotrexate 40 mg/m^2 I.V. on days 1 and 8

5-Fluorouracil (5-FU) 600 mg/m^2 I.V. on days 1 and 8

Repeat cycle every 28 days.

Patients older than age 60:

Cyclophosphamide 100 mg/m^2 P.O. on days 1 through 14

Methotrexate 30 mg/m^2 I.V. on days 1 and 8

5-FU 400 mg/m^2 I.V. on days 1 and 8

Repeat cycle every 28 days.

Reference: Bonadonna G, et al. *N Engl J Med.* 1976;294:405-410; Bonadonna G, et al. *N Engl J Med.* 1995;332:901-906; Amadori D, et al. *J Clin Oncol.* 2000;18:3125-3134.

Supportive therapy

Patients are at moderate to high risk for nausea and vomiting, anemia, and neutropenia. Supportive and/or prophylactic therapies are recommended.

Docetaxel

Docetaxel 60 to 100 mg/m^2 I.V. over 1 hour on day 1

Repeat every 21 days.

Reference: Nabholtz J-M, et al. *J Clin Oncol.* 1999;17:1413-1424; docetaxel prescribing information.

Supportive therapy

Patients are at moderate to high risk for nausea and vomiting, anemia, neutropenia, diarrhea, and hypersensitivity reactions. Supportive and/or prophylactic therapies are recommended.

FAC (or CAF) (5-fluorouracil, doxorubicin [Adriamycin], cyclophosphamide)

5-Fluorouracil (5-FU) 500 mg/m^2 I.V. on day 1

Doxorubicin 50 mg/m^2 I.V. on day 1

Cyclophosphamide 500 mg/m^2 I.V. on day 1

Repeat cycle every 21 days.

Or

Cyclophosphamide 600 mg/m^2 I.V. on day 1
Doxorubicin 60 mg/m^2 I.V. on day 1
5-FU 600 mg/m^2 I.V. on days 1 and 8
Repeat cycle every 28 days.

Reference: Stewart DJ, et al. *J Clin Oncol.* 1997;15:1897-1905; Budman DR, et al. *J Natl Cancer Inst.* 1998;90:1205-1211.

Supportive therapy

Patients are at moderate to high risk for nausea and vomiting, anemia, neutropenia, diarrhea, and constipation. Supportive and/or prophylactic therapies are recommended.

FEC-100 (5-fluorouracil, epirubicin, cyclophosphamide)

5-Fluorouracil 500 mg/m^2 I.V. on day 1
Epirubicin 100 mg/m^2 I.V. on day 1
Cyclophosphamide 500 mg/m^2 I.V. on day 1
Repeat cycle every 21 days.

Reference: French Epirubicin Study Group. *J Clin Oncol.* 200;18:3115-3124.

Supportive therapy

Patients are at moderate to high risk for nausea and vomiting, anemia, neutropenia, and diarrhea. Supportive and/or prophylactic therapies are recommended.

GT (gemcitabine, paclitaxel [Taxol])

Paclitaxel 175 mg/m^2 I.V. over 3 hours on day 1 only before gemcitabine
Gemcitabine 1,250 mg/m^2 I.V. over 30 minutes on days 1 and 8
Repeat cycle every 21 days.

Reference: Albain K, et al. *ASCO.* 2004;23:Abstract #510.

Supportive therapy

Patients are at moderate to high risk for nausea and vomiting, anemia, neutropenia, and hypersensitivity reactions. Supportive and/or prophylactic therapies are recommended.

Paclitaxel

Paclitaxel 175 or 250 mg/m^2 I.V. over 3 hours on day 1

Repeat every 21 days.
Or
Paclitaxel 80 mg/m^2 I.V. over 1 hour on day 1
Repeat every 7 days.

Reference: Seidman AD, et al. *J Clin Oncol.* 1995;13:2575-2581; Smith RE, et al. *J Clin Oncol.* 1999;17:3403-3411; *Breast cancer.* NCCN Practice Guidelines in Oncology, 2005.

Supportive therapy

Patients are at moderate to high risk for nausea and vomiting, anemia, neutropenia, diarrhea, and hypersensitivity reactions. Supportive and/or prophylactic therapies are recommended.

Trastuzumab, vinorelbine

Trastuzumab 4 mg/kg I.V. over 90 minutes on day 1 of first cycle. Give 2 mg/kg I.V. over 30 minutes in subsequent cycles.
Vinorelbine 25 mg/m^2 I.V. over 6 to 10 minutes (given after trastuzumab). Follow with 125 ml of saline I.V.
Repeat cycle every 7 days.

Reference: Burstein HJ, et al. *J Clin Oncol.* 2001;19:2722-2730; Burstein HJ, et al. *J Clin Oncol.* 2003;21:2889-2895.

Supportive therapy

Patients are at moderate to high risk for nausea and vomiting, anemia, neutropenia, and diarrhea. Supportive and/or prophylactic therapies are recommended.

Cervical cancer

Cisplatin

Cisplatin 50 to 100 mg/m^2 I.V. on day 1
Repeat every 21 days.

Reference: Bonomi P, et al. *J Clin Oncol.* 1985;3(8):1079-1085.

Supportive therapy

Patients are at moderate to high risk for nausea and vomiting, anemia, neutropenia, diarrhea, and cisplatin-induced nephrotoxicity. Supportive and/or prophylactic therapies are recommended.

Cisplatin, paclitaxel

Paclitaxel 135 mg/m^2 I.V. over 24 hours on day 1
Cisplatin 50 mg/m^2 I.V. on day 2
Repeat cycle every 21 days.

Reference: Moore DH, et al. *J Clin Oncol.* 2004;22:3113-3119.

Supportive therapy

Patients are at moderate to high risk for nausea and vomiting, anemia, neutropenia, diarrhea, hypersensitivity reactions, and cisplatin-induced nephrotoxicity. Supportive and/or prophylactic therapies are recommended.

Cisplatin, topotecan

Cisplatin 50 mg/m^2 I.V. on day 1
Topotecan 0.75 mg/m^2 I.V. on days 1 through 3
Repeat cycle every 21 days.

Reference: Long HJ, et al. *J Clin Oncol.* 2005;23:4626-4633.

Supportive therapy

Patients are at moderate to high risk for nausea and vomiting, anemia, neutropenia, diarrhea, and cisplatin-induced nephrotoxicity. Supportive and/or prophylactic therapies are recommended.

Docetaxel

Docetaxel 100 mg/m^2 I.V. over 1 hour on day 1
Repeat every 21 days.

Reference: Vallejo CT, et al. *Am J Clin Oncol.* 2003;26:477-482.

Supportive therapy

Patients are at moderate to high risk for nausea and vomiting, anemia, neutropenia, and hypersensitivity reactions. Supportive and/or prophylactic therapies are recommended.

Gemcitabine, cisplatin

Cisplatin 50 mg/m^2 I.V. over 30 minutes on day 1
Gemcitabine 1,250 mg/m^2 I.V. over 30 minutes on days 1 and 8
Repeat cycle every 21 days.

Reference: Burnett AF, et al. *Gynecol Oncol.* 2000;76:63-66.

Supportive therapy

Patients are at moderate to high risk for nausea and vomiting, anemia, neutropenia, diarrhea, and cisplatin-induced nephrotoxicity. Supportive and/or prophylactic therapies are recommended.

Paclitaxel

Paclitaxel 170 mg/m^2 I.V. over 24 hours on day 1
Repeat every 21 days.

Reference: Curtin JP, et al. *J Clin Oncol.* 2001;19:1275-1278.

Supportive therapy

Patients are at moderate to high risk for nausea and vomiting, anemia, neutropenia, and hypersensitivity reactions. Supportive and/or prophylactic therapies are recommended.

Chronic myelogenous leukemia

Imatinib mesylate

Imatinib 400 mg/day P.O. (chronic phase) daily
Or
Imatinib 600 mg/day P.O. (accelerated phase blast crisis) daily
Continue treatment until disease progresses.

Reference: O'Brien SG, et al. *N Engl J Med.* 2003;348:994-1004; Talpaz M, et. al. *Blood.* 2002;99:1928-1937.

Supportive therapy

Patients are at moderate to high risk for nausea and vomiting and diarrhea. Supportive and/or prophylactic therapies are recommended.

Interferon alfa-2b, cytarabine

Interferon alfa-2b increased as tolerated to target dosage of 5 million units/m^2 subcutaneously daily
Cytarabine 20 mg/m^2 subcutaneously daily for 10 days (maximum daily dosage, 40 mg). Start cytarabine once tolerated dosage of interferon is achieved.
Repeat cytarabine cycle monthly.

Reference: O'Brien SG, et al. *N Engl J Med.* 2003;348:994-1004.

See appendices for supportive therapies.

Supportive therapy

Patients are at moderate to high risk for nausea and vomiting, neutropenia, and diarrhea. Supportive and/or prophylactic therapies are recommended.

CNS tumors

Carmustine

Carmustine 200 mg/m^2 I.V. as single dose
Repeat every 6 to 8 weeks.

Reference: Selker RG, et al. *Neurosurgery.* 2002;51:343-355.

Supportive therapy

Patients are at moderate to high risk for nausea and vomiting, anemia, and neutropenia. Supportive and/or prophylactic therapies are recommended.

Temozolomide

Temozolomide 200 mg/m^2 P.O. daily (chemotherapy naive) *or* 150 mg/m^2 P.O. daily (prior chemotherapy) on days 1 through 5
Repeat every 28 days.

Reference: Yung WK. *J Clin Oncol.* 1999;17:2762-2771.

Supportive therapy

Patients are at moderate to high risk for nausea and vomiting and neutropenia. Supportive and/or prophylactic therapies are recommended.

Colon, rectal, and anal cancers

Bolus or infusional 5-fluorouracil, leucovorin

Mayo

5-Fluorouracil (5-FU) 425 mg/m^2 daily by I.V. bolus 1 hour after start of leucovorin on days 1 through 5
Leucovorin 20 mg/m^2 daily by I.V. bolus on days 1 through 5
Repeat cycle in 4 weeks and 8 weeks, then every 5 weeks.

Reference: Poon MA, et al. *J Clin Oncol.* 1991;11:1967.

Roswell Park

5-FU 600 mg/m^2 by I.V. bolus 1 hour after start of leucovorin on days 1, 8, 15, 22, 29, 36

Leucovorin 500 mg/m^2 I.V. over 2 hours on days 1, 8, 15, 22, 29, 36

Repeat cycle every 8 weeks.

Reference: Petrelli N, et al. *J Clin Oncol.* 1987;5:1559-1565.

de Gramont

5-FU Initial dose, 400 mg/m^2 by I.V. bolus, then 600 mg/m^2 by continuous I.V. infusion over 22 hours on days 1 and 2 every 2 weeks

Leucovorin 200 mg/m^2 daily I.V. over 2 hours on days 1 and 2 every 2 weeks (before 5-FU)

References: de Gramont A, et al. *J Clin Oncol.* 1997;15:808-815; de Gramont A, et al. *J Clin Oncol.* 2000;18:2938-2947.

Supportive therapy

Patients are at moderate to high risk for nausea and vomiting, anemia, and diarrhea. Supportive and/or prophylactic therapies are recommended.

Capecitabine

Capecitabine 2,500 mg/m^2 P.O. daily in two divided doses on days 1 through 14

Repeat every 21 days.

Reference: Scherthauer W, et al. *Annals Oncol.* 2003;14:1735-1743.

Supportive therapy

Patients are at moderate to high risk for nausea and vomiting, anemia, and diarrhea. Supportive and/or prophylactic therapies are recommended.

Cetuximab, irinotecan

Cetuximab Initial dose, 400 mg/ m^2 I.V. over 120 minutes, then 250 mg/m^2 I.V. over 60 minutes weekly

Irinotecan 350 mg/m^2 I.V. over 90 minutes

Repeat cycle every 21 days.

Or

Cetuximab Initial dose, 400 mg/ m^2 I.V. over 120 minutes, then 250 mg/m^2 I.V. over 60 minutes weekly

Irinotecan 180 mg/m^2 I.V. over 90 minutes

Repeat cycle every 14 days.

Reference: Cunningham D, et al. *N Engl J Med.* 2004;351:337-345.

Supportive therapy

Patients are at moderate to high risk for nausea and vomiting, anemia, neutropenia, diarrhea, and hypersensitivity reactions. Supportive and/or prophylactic therapies are recommended.

5-Fluorouracil, leucovorin, oxaliplatin combinations

FOLFOX4
Oxaliplatin 85 mg/m^2 I.V. over 2 hours on day 1
Leucovorin 200 mg/m^2 I.V. over 2 hours (on days 1 and 2); then
5-Fluorouracil (5-FU) 400 mg/m^2 by I.V. bolus, followed by 600 mg/m^2 by continuous I.V. infusion over 22 hours on days 1 and 2
Repeat cycle every 14 days.

FOLFOX6
Oxaliplatin 100 mg/m^2 I.V. over 2 hours on day 1
Leucovorin 400 mg/m^2 I.V. over 2 hours (on days 1 and 2); then
5-FU 400 mg/m^2 by I.V. bolus, followed by 2,400 mg/m^2 by continuous I.V. infusion over 46 hours
Repeat cycle every 14 days. If no toxicity greater than grade 1 occurs after first two cycles, increase 5-FU dosage to 3,000 mg/m^2.

mFOLFOX6
Oxaliplatin 85 mg/m^2 I.V. over 2 hours on day 1
Leucovorin 400 mg/m^2 I.V. over 2 hours on days 1 and 2; then
5-FU 400 mg/m^2 by I.V. bolus, followed by 2,400 mg/m^2 by continuous I.V. infusion over 46 hours
Repeat cycle every 14 days. If no toxicity greater than grade 1 occurs after first two cycles, increase 5-FU dosage to 3,000 mg/m^2.

FOLFOX7
Oxaliplatin 130 mg/m^2 I.V. over 2 hours on day 1
Leucovorin 400 mg/m^2 I.V. over 2 hours on days 1 and 2; then
5-FU 400 mg/m^2 by I.V. bolus, followed by 2,400 mg/m^2 by continuous I.V. infusion over 46 to 48 hours
Repeat cycle every 14 days. If no toxicity greater than grade 1 occurs after first two cycles, increase 5-FU dosage to 3,000 mg/m^2.

References: Colucci G, et al. *J Clin Oncol.* 2005;23:4866-4875; Tournigand C, et al. *J Clin Oncol.* 2004;22:229-237; Cheeseman SL, et al. *Br J*

Cancer. 2002;87:393-399; Maindrault-Goebel F, et al. *Euro J Cancer*. 2002;37:1000-1005.

Supportive therapy

Patients are at moderate to high risk for nausea and vomiting, anemia, neutropenia, and diarrhea. Supportive and/or prophylactic therapies are recommended.

IFL/BV (irinotecan, 5-fluorouracil, leucovorin, bevacizumab)

Irinotecan 125 mg/m^2 I.V. over 90 minutes on days 1, 8, 15, and 22
Leucovorin 20 mg/m^2 daily by I.V. bolus on days 1, 8, 15, 22
5-Fluorouracil 500 mg/m^2 daily by I.V. bolus on days 1, 8, 15, and 22
Bevacizumab 5 mg/kg I.V. over 90 minutes, then decrease to 30 to 60 minutes, if tolerated, every 14 days
Repeat cycle every 6 weeks.

Reference: Hurwitz H, et al. *N Engl J Med*. 2004;350:2335-2342.

Supportive therapy

Patients are at moderate to high risk for nausea and vomiting, anemia, neutropenia, and diarrhea. Supportive and/or prophylactic therapies are recommended.

Irinotecan, leucovorin, 5-fluorouracil combinations

Douillard
Irinotecan 180 mg/m^2 I.V. over 2 hours on day 1
Leucovorin 200 mg/m^2 I.V. over 2 hours on days 1 and 2
5-Fluorouracil (5-FU) Initial dose, 400 mg/m^2 by I.V. bolus, then 600 mg/m^2 by continuous I.V. infusion over next 22 hours on days 1 and 2. Start 5-FU after leucovorin.
Repeat cycle every 14 days.

FOLFIRI
Irinotecan 180 mg/m^2 I.V. over 90 minutes on day 1
Leucovorin 400 mg/m^2 I.V. over 2 hours during irinotecan infusion
5-FU Initial dose, 400 mg/m^2 by I.V. bolus, then 2,400 mg/m^2 by continuous I.V. infusion over next 46 hours. Start 5-FU after leucovorin.
Repeat cycle every 14 days.

IFL (Saltz)
Irinotecan 125 mg/m^2 I.V. over 90 minutes on days 1, 8, 15, and 22

Leucovorin 20 mg/m^2 by I.V. bolus on days 1, 8, 15, and 22
5-FU 500 mg/m^2 I.V. bolus on days 1, 8, 15, and 22
Repeat cycle every 6 weeks.

Reference: Douillard JY, et al. *Lancet.* 2000;355:1041-1047; Tourigand C, et al. *J Clin Oncol.* 2004;22:229-237; Saltz LB, et al. *N Engl J Med.* 2000;343:905-914.

Supportive therapy

Patients are at moderate to high risk for nausea and vomiting, anemia, neutropenia, and diarrhea. Supportive and/or prophylactic therapies are recommended.

XELOX (capecitabine [Xeloda], oxaliplatin)

Oxaliplatin 130 mg/m^2 I.V. over 2 hours on day 1
Capecitabine 1,000 mg/m^2 P.O. twice daily from evening of day 1 to morning of day 15
Repeat cycle every 21 days.

Reference: Makatsoris T, et al. *Int J Gastro Cancer.* 2005;35:103-109; Cassidy J, et al. *J Clin Oncol.* 2004;22:2084-2091.

Supportive therapy

Patients are at moderate to high risk for nausea and vomiting, anemia, neutropenia, and diarrhea. Supportive and/or prophylactic therapies are recommended.

Esophageal cancer

Cisplatin, 5-fluorouracil

Cisplatin 75 mg/m^2 I.V. on day 1 of weeks 1, 5, 8, and 11
5-Fluorouracil (5-FU) 1,000 mg/m^2 daily by continuous I.V. infusion on days 1 through 4 of weeks 1, 5, 8, and 11
Radiation therapy 50 Gy in 25 fractions over 5 weeks

Reference: Cooper JS, et al. *JAMA.* 1999;281:1623-1627.
Or
Cisplatin 75 mg/m^2 by I.V. bolus over 30 minutes on day 1
5-FU 1,000 mg/m^2 by continuous I.V. infusion on days 1 through 4
Radiation therapy 1.8 Gy/day, 5 days a week of weeks 1 through 5 or weeks 1 through 7

Repeat cycle after 4-week rest from radiation (week 9).

Reference: Minsky BD, et al. *J Clin Oncol.* 2002;20:1167-1174.

Or

5-FU 15 mg/kg I.V. over 16 hours on days 1 through 5
Cisplatin 75 mg/m^2 I.V. over 8 hours on day 7 of weeks 1 and 6
Radiation therapy 40 Gy in 15 fractions over 3 weeks, beginning concurrently with first course of chemotherapy
Repeat cycle in 6 weeks.

Reference: Walsh TN, et al. *N Engl J Med.* 1996;335:462-467.

Or

Cisplatin 80 mg/m^2 I.V. over 4 hours on day 1
5-FU 1,000 mg/m^2 by continuous I.V. infusion daily for 4 days, followed by surgical resection after 2 cycles
Repeat cycle every 21 days.

Reference: Medical Research Council Oesophageal Cancer Working Group. *Lancet.* 2002;359:1727-1733.

Supportive therapy

Patients are at moderate to high risk for nausea and vomiting, anemia, neutropenia, diarrhea, and cisplatin-induced nephrotoxicity. Supportive and/or prophylactic therapies are recommended.

Cisplatin, paclitaxel

Cisplatin 75 mg/m^2 I.V. over 2 hours on day 1
Paclitaxel 60 mg/m^2 I.V. over 3 hours on days 1, 8, 15, and 22
Radiation therapy 1.5 Gy twice daily on days 1 to 5, 8 to 12, and 15 through 19

Reference: Urba SG, et al. *Cancer.* 2003;98:2177-2183.

Supportive therapy

Patients are at moderate to high risk for nausea and vomiting, anemia, neutropenia, hypersensitivity reactions, and cisplatin-induced nephrotoxicity. Supportive and/or prophylactic therapies are recommended.

CPT-11 + CDDP (irinotecan + cisplatin)

Irinotecan 65 mg/m^2 I.V. over 90 minutes on days 1, 8, 15, and 22
Cisplatin 30 mg/m^2 I.V. over 2 hours on days 1, 8, 15, and 22

After 2-week rest, repeat cycle every 6 weeks.

Or

Irinotecan 65 mg/m^2 I.V. over 90 minutes on days 1 and 8
Cisplatin 30 mg/m^2 I.V. over 2 hours on days 1 and 8
After 1-week rest, repeat cycle every 21 days.

Reference: Ilson DH, et al. *J Clin Oncol.* 1999;17:3270-3275; Ilson DH. *Oncology.* 2004;18(14):22-25.

Supportive therapy

Patients are at moderate to high risk for nausea and vomiting, neutropenia, diarrhea, and cisplatin-induced nephrotoxicity. Supportive and/or prophylactic therapies are recommended.

Paclitaxel

Paclitaxel 250 mg/m^2 by I.V. infusion over 24 hours on day 1 only
Repeat every 21 days.

Reference: Ajani JA, et al. *J Natl Cancer Inst.* 1994;86:1086-1091; Ajani JA, et al. *Semin Oncol.* 1996;(5, Suppl 12):S55-S58.

Supportive therapy

Patients are at moderate to high risk for nausea and vomiting, anemia, neutropenia, and hypersensitivity reactions. Supportive and/or prophylactic therapies are recommended.

Paclitaxel, cisplatin, 5-fluorouracil

Paclitaxel 175 mg/m^2 by I.V. infusion over 3 hours on day 1
Cisplatin 20 mg/m^2 I.V. daily on days 1 through 5 for first three cycles; 15 mg/m^2 I.V. daily on days 1 through 5 from cycle 4 on
5-Fluorouracil 750 mg/m^2 by continuous I.V. infusion on days 1 through 5
Repeat cycle every 28 days.

Reference: Ilson DH, et al. *J Clin Oncol.* 1998;16:1826-1834.

Supportive therapy

Patients are at moderate to high risk for nausea and vomiting, anemia, neutropenia, diarrhea, hypersensitivity reactions, and cisplatin-induced nephrotoxicity. Supportive and/or prophylactic therapies are recommended.

Gastric cancer

DCF (or TCF) (docetaxel [Taxotere], cisplatin, 5-fluorouracil)

Docetaxel 85 mg/m^2 I.V. on day 1
Cisplatin 75 mg/m^2 I.V. on day 1
5-Fluorouracil 300 mg/m^2 by continuous I.V. infusion on days 1 through 14
Repeat cycle every 21 days for maximum of eight cycles.

Reference: Roth D, et al. *J Clin Oncol.* 2004;22(14S):4020.

Supportive therapy
Patients are at moderate to high risk for nausea and vomiting, anemia, neutropenia, diarrhea, hypersensitivity reactions, and cisplatin-induced nephrotoxicity. Supportive and/or prophylactic therapies are recommended.

ECF (epirubicin, cisplatin, 5-fluorouracil)

Epirubicin 50 mg/m^2 by I.V. bolus on day 1, *Cisplatin* 60 mg/m^2 I.V. over 2 hours on day 1
5-Fluorouracil 200 mg/m^2 daily by continuous I.V. infusion on days 1 through 21
Repeat cycle every 21 to 28 days.

Reference: Waters JS, et al. *Br J Cancer.* 1999;80:269-272; Webb A, et al. *J Clin Oncol.* 1997;15:261-267; Findlay M, et al. *Ann Oncol.* 1994;5:609-616.

Supportive therapy
Patients are at moderate to high risk for nausea and vomiting, anemia, neutropenia, diarrhea, and cisplatin-induced nephrotoxicity. Supportive and/or prophylactic therapies are recommended.

ELF (etoposide, leucovorin, 5-fluorouracil)

Leucovorin 150 mg/m^2 I.V. daily over 10 minutes on days 1 through 3, then
Etoposide 120 mg/m^2 I.V. daily over 30 minutes on days 1 through 3, then

5-Fluorouracil (5-FU) 500 mg/m^2 I.V. daily over 10 minutes on days 1 through 3

Repeat cycle every 21 days. Or

Leucovorin 300 mg/m^2 I.V. daily over 10 minutes on days 1 through 3, then

Etoposide 120 mg/m^2 I.V. daily over 50 minutes on days 1 through 3, then

5-FU 500 mg/m^2 daily by I.V. bolus over 10 minutes on days 1 through 3

Repeat cycle every 21 days.

Reference: di Bartolomeo M, et al. *Oncology.* 1995;52:41-44; Vanhoefer U, et al. *J Clin Oncol.* 2000;18:2648-2657; Moehler M, et al. *Br J Cancer.* 2005;92:2122-2128; Wilke H. *Cancer Treat Res.* 1991;55:363-373.

Supportive therapy

Patients are at moderate to high risk for nausea and vomiting, anemia, neutropenia, and diarrhea. Supportive and/or prophylactic therapies are recommended.

FAMTX (5-fluorouracil, doxorubicin [Adriamycin], methotrexate)

Methotrexate 1,500 mg/m^2 I.V. on day 1

5-Fluorouracil 1,500 mg/m^2 I.V. on day 1 given 1 hour after methotrexate dose

Leucovorin 15 mg/m^2 P.O. given 24 hours after methotrexate dose and every 6 hours for 48 hours

Doxorubicin 30 mg/m^2 I.V., day 15

Repeat cycle every 28 days.

Reference: Wills J, et al. *J Clin Oncol.* 1986;4:1799-1803; Vanhoefer U, et al. *J Clin Oncol.* 2000;18:2648-2657.

Supportive therapy

Patients are at moderate to high risk for nausea and vomiting, anemia, neutropenia, diarrhea, and methotrexate-induced nephrotoxicity. Supportive and/or prophylactic therapies are recommended.

FOLFOX6 (oxaliplatin, leucovorin, 5-fluorouracil)

Oxaliplatin 100 mg/m^2 I.V. on day 1

Leucovorin 400 mg/m^2 I.V. over 2 hours on day 1, followed by

5-Fluorouracil (5-FU) Initial dose, 400 mg/m^2 I.V. on day 1, then 3,000 mg/m^2 by continuous I.V. infusion over next 46 hours
Repeat cycle every 14 days.

Reference: Louvet C, et al. *J Clin Oncol.* 2002;20:4543-4548.

Supportive therapy

Patients are at moderate to high risk for nausea and vomiting, anemia, neutropenia, and diarrhea. Supportive and/or prophylactic therapies are recommended.

TC (docetaxel [Taxotere], cisplatin)

Docetaxel 85 mg/m^2 I.V. over 1 hour on day 1 followed by
Cisplatin 75 mg/m^2 I.V. over 1 hour on day 1
Repeat cycle every 21 days for maximum of eight cycles.

Reference: Roth AD, et al. *Ann Oncol.* 2000;11:301-306.

Supportive therapy

Patients are at moderate to high risk for nausea and vomiting, anemia, neutropenia, hypersensitivity reactions, and cisplatin-induced nephrotoxicity. Supportive and/or prophylactic therapies are recommended.

Head and neck cancers

Cisplatin, 5-fluorouracil

Cisplatin 100 mg/m^2 by continuous I.V. infusion over 24 hours on day 1
5-Fluorouracil (5-FU) 5,000 mg/m^2 by continuous I.V. infusion over 120 hours on days 1 through 5
Repeat cycle every 21 days.

Reference: DeAndres L, et al. *J Clin Oncol.* 1995;13:1493-1500.
Or
Cisplatin 100 mg/m^2 I.V. over 1 hour on days 1 and 29
5-FU 1,000 mg/m^2 on days 1 through 4 and 29 through 32. Both drugs given in combination with radiation.
Give for one cycle.

Reference: Poole ME, et al. *Arch Otolaryngol Head Neck Surg.* 2001;127:1446-1450.

See appendices for supportive therapies.

Or

Cisplatin 100 mg/m^2 by I.V. infusion on day 1

5-FU 1,000 mg/m^2 I.V. over 120 hours. Both drugs given in combination with radiation.

Give for three cycles.

Reference: Lewin F, et al. *Radiother Oncol.* 1997;43:23-28.

Supportive therapy

Patients are at moderate to high risk for nausea and vomiting, anemia, neutropenia, diarrhea, and cisplatin-induced nephrotoxicity. Supportive and/or prophylactic therapies are recommended.

Hepatobiliary cancer

5-Fluorouracil, leucovorin

Leucovorin 25 mg/m^2 daily by I.V. infusion over 2 hours on days 1 through 5

5-Fluorouracil 375 mg/m^2 daily by I.V. infusion on days 1 through 5

Repeat cycle every 21 to 28 days.

Reference: Choi CW. *Am J Clin Oncol.* 2000;23:425-428.

Supportive therapy

Patients are at moderate to high risk for nausea and vomiting, anemia, and diarrhea. Supportive and/or prophylactic therapies are recommended.

Gemcitabine

Gemcitabine 1,000 mg/m^2 I.V. over 30 minutes for 3 weeks

Repeat every 28 days.

Reference: Kubicka S, et al. *Hepatogastroenterology.* 2001;48:783-789.

Supportive therapy

Patients are at moderate to high risk for nausea and vomiting and anemia. Supportive and/or prophylactic therapies are recommended.

Hodgkin's disease

ABVD (doxorubicin [Adriamycin], bleomycin, vinblastine, dacarbazine)

Doxorubicin 25 mg/m^2 I.V. on days 1 and 15
Bleomycin 10 units/m^2 I.V. on days 1 and 15
Vinblastine 6 mg/m^2 I.V. on days 1 and 15
Dacarbazine (DTIC) 375 mg/m^2 I.V. on days 1 and 15
Repeat cycle every 28 days.

Reference: Bonadonna G, et al. *Am Soc Clin Oncol.* 2004;22:2835-2841.

Supportive therapy

Patients are at moderate to high risk for nausea and vomiting, anemia, neutropenia, and diarrhea. Supportive and/or prophylactic therapies are recommended.

BEACOPP (bleomycin, etoposide, doxorubicin [Adriamycin], cyclophosphamide, vincristine [Oncovin], procarbazine, prednisone)

Bleomycin 10 mg/m^2 I.V. on day 8
Etoposide 100 mg/m^2 I.V. on days 1 through 3
Doxorubicin 25 mg/m^2 I.V. on day 1
Cyclophosphamide 650 mg/m^2 I.V. on day 1
Vincristine 1.4 mg/m^2 I.V. on day 1 or day 8
Procarbazine 100 mg/m^2 P.O. on days 1 through 7
Prednisone 40 mg/m^2 P.O. on days 1 through 14
Repeat cycle every 21 days.

Reference: Tesch H, et al. Blood. 1998;92:4560-4567; Pazdur R, et al., eds. *Cancer Management: A Multidisciplinary Approach.* 9th ed. Lawrence, KS: CMP Media; 2005.

Supportive therapy

Patients are at moderate to high risk for nausea and vomiting, anemia, neutropenia, diarrhea, and constipation. Supportive and/or prophylactic therapies are recommended.

Stanford V (doxorubicin, vinblastine, mechlorethamine, vincristine, bleomycin, etoposide, prednisone)

Doxorubicin 25 mg/m^2 I.V. on days 1 and 15

Vinblastine 6 mg/m^2 I.V. on days 1 and 15

Mechlorethamine 6 mg/m^2 I.V. on day 1

Vincristine 1.4 mg/m^2 I.V. on days 8 and 22

Bleomycin 5 units/m^2 I.V. on days 8 and 22

Etoposide 60 mg/m^2 I.V. on days 15 and 16

Prednisone 40 mg/m^2 P.O. every other day for 10 weeks; then taper dosage downward by 10 mg every other day.

Repeat chemotherapy agents every 28 days for three cycles. Give prednisone continuously for 10 weeks, then taper as noted above.

Reference: Horning SJ, et al. *J Clin Oncol.* 2002;20:630-637; Pazdur R, et al., eds. *Cancer Management. A Multidisciplinary Approach.* 9th ed. Lawrence, KS: CMP Media; 2005.

Supportive therapy

Patients are at moderate to high risk for nausea and vomiting, anemia, neutropenia, diarrhea, and constipation. Supportive and/or prophylactic therapies are recommended.

Kidney cancer

Interferon alfa-2a, interleukin-2

Interleukin-2 (IL-2) 18 million units/m^2 daily by continuous I.V. infusion on days 1 through 5; repeat after 6 days of rest (induction), followed 3 weeks later by 18 million units/m^2 daily by continuous I.V. infusion on days 1 through 5 (maintenance).

Repeat maintenance cycle for four cycles, with 3 weeks' rest after each cycle.

Interferon alfa-2a 6 million units subcutaneously three times per week during each IL-2 cycle (induction and maintenance)

Reference: Negrier S, et al. *N Engl J Med.* 1998;338:1273-1278; Dutcher JP, et al. *Cancer J Sci Am.* 1997;3:157-162.

Supportive therapy

Patients are at moderate to high risk for nausea and vomiting, diarrhea, flulike symptoms, and infection. Supportive and/or prophylactic therapies are recommended.

Interleukin-2

High dose:

Interleukin-2 (IL-2) 600,000 to 720,000 units/kg I.V. over 15 minutes every 8 hours until toxicity occurs or 14 doses have been given over 5 days, followed by 7 to 10 days of rest.

Repeat cycle twice.

Low dose:

IL-2 Give 72,000 units/kg I.V. over 15 minutes every 8 hours until toxicity occurs or 14 doses have been given over 5 days; follow by 7 to 10 days of rest.

Repeat cycle up to three times.

Or

IL-2 Give 3 million units/m^2 daily by continuous I.V. infusion on days 1 through 5 and 12 through 17

Repeat second cycle every 28 days for four cycles.

Reference: Fyfe G, et al. *J Clin Oncol.* 1995;13:688-696; Pazdur R (ed), et al. *Cancer Management: A Multidisciplinary Approach.* 8th ed. CMP Healthcare Media; 2005; Yang JC, et al. *J Clin Oncol.* 2003;21:3127-3132.

Supportive therapy

Patients are at moderate to high risk for nausea and vomiting, diarrhea, flulike symptoms, and infection. Supportive and/or prophylactic therapies are recommended.

Lung cancer (non-small-cell)

Carboplatin, paclitaxel

Carboplatin to AUC of 5 or 6 I.V. on day 1
Paclitaxel 175 to 225 mg/m^2 I.V. over 3 hours on day 1

Repeat cycle every 21 days.

Reference: Strauss GM. *J Clin Oncol.* 2004;22(14S):7019.

Supportive therapy

Patients are at moderate to high risk for nausea and vomiting, anemia, neutropenia, diarrhea, constipation, and hypersensitivity reactions. Supportive and/or prophylactic therapies are recommended.

Cisplatin, docetaxel

Cisplatin 75 mg/m² I.V. on day 1
Docetaxel 75 mg/m² I.V. on day 1
Repeat cycle every 21 days.

Reference: Fossella F, et al. *Am Soc Clin Oncol.* 2003;21:3016-3024.

Supportive therapy

Patients are at moderate to high risk for nausea and vomiting, anemia, neutropenia, diarrhea, hypersensitivity reactions, and cisplatin-induced nephrotoxicity. Supportive and/or prophylactic therapies are recommended.

Cisplatin, gemcitabine

Cisplatin 100 mg/m² I.V. on day 1
Gemcitabine 1,200 mg/m² I.V. on days 1 and 8
Repeat cycle every 21 days.

Reference: Gridelli C, et al. *Am Soc Clin Oncol.* 2003;21:3025-3034.
Or
Gemcitabine 1,000 mg/m² I.V. on days 1, 8, and 15
Cisplatin 100 mg/m² I.V. on day 2
Repeat cycle every 28 days.

Reference: Crino L, et al. *J Clin Oncol.* 1999;17:3522-3530.

Supportive therapy

Patients are at moderate to high risk for nausea and vomiting, anemia, neutropenia, diarrhea, constipation, and cisplatin-induced nephrotoxicity. Supportive and/or prophylactic therapies are recommended.

Cisplatin, paclitaxel

Cisplatin 80 mg/m² I.V. over 30 minutes on day 1
Paclitaxel 175 mg/m² I.V. over 3 hours on day 1
Repeat cycle every 21 days.

Reference: Gatzemeier U. *J Clin Oncol.* 2000;18:3390-3399.

Supportive therapy

Patients are at moderate to high risk for nausea and vomiting, anemia, neutropenia, diarrhea, hypersensitivity reactions, and cisplatin-induced nephrotoxicity. Supportive and/or prophylactic therapies are recommended.

Docetaxel

Docetaxel 100 mg/m^2 I.V. over 1 hour on day 1
Or
Docetaxel 75 mg/m^2 I.V. over 1 hour on day 1
Repeat every 21 days.

Reference: Gandara DR, et al. *J Clin Oncol.* 2000;18:131-135; Fossella FV, et al. *J Clin Oncol.* 2000;18:2354-2362.

Supportive therapy

Patients are at moderate to high risk for nausea and vomiting, anemia, neutropenia, and hypersensitivity reactions. Supportive and/or prophylactic therapies are recommended.

Erlotinib

Erlotinib 150 mg P.O. daily 2 hours after ingestion of food. Continue treatment until disease progresses or unacceptable toxicity occurs.

Reference: Pérez-Soler R. *J Clin Oncol.* 2004;22:3238-3247.

Supportive therapy

Patients are at moderate to high risk for nausea and vomiting and diarrhea. Supportive and/or prophylactic therapies are recommended.

Gemcitabine, docetaxel

Gemcitabine 1,000 mg/m^2 I.V. on days 1 and 8
Docetaxel 100 mg/m^2 I.V. on day 8
Repeat cycle every 21 days.

Reference: Georgoulias V, et al. *J Clin Oncol.* 2005;23:2937-2945.

Supportive therapy

Patients are at moderate to high risk for nausea and vomiting, anemia, neutropenia, diarrhea, constipation, and hypersensitivity reactions. Supportive and/or prophylactic therapies are recommended.

See appendices for supportive therapies.

Gemcitabine, paclitaxel

Gemcitabine 1,000 mg/m^2 I.V. on days 1 and 8
Paclitaxel 200 mg/m^2 I.V. over 3 hours on day 1
Repeat cycle every 21 days.

Reference: Kosmidis P, et al. *J Clin Oncol.* 2002;20:3578-3585.

Supportive therapy

Patients are at moderate to high risk for nausea and vomiting, anemia, neutropenia, diarrhea, constipation, and hypersensitivity reactions. Supportive and/or prophylactic therapies are recommended.

Gemcitabine, vinorelbine

Gemcitabine 1,200 mg/m^2 I.V. on days 1 and 8
Vinorelbine 30 mg/m^2 I.V. on days 1 and 8
Repeat cycle every 21 days.
Or
Gemcitabine 800 to 1,000 mg/m^2 I.V. on days 1, 8, and 15
Vinorelbine 20 mg/m^2 I.V. on days 1, 8, and 15
Repeat cycle every 28 days.

Reference: Frasci G, et al. *J Clin Oncol.* 2000;18:2529-2536; Chen YM, et al. *Chest.* 2000;117:1583-1589; Hainsworth JD, et al. *Cancer.* 2000;88:1353-1358.

Supportive therapy

Patients are at moderate to high risk for nausea and vomiting, anemia, neutropenia, diarrhea, and constipation. Supportive and/or prophylactic therapies are recommended.

Lung cancer (small-cell)

CAE (or ACE) (cyclophosphamide, doxorubicin [Adriamycin], etoposide)

Cyclophosphamide 1,000 mg/m^2 I.V. on day 1
Doxorubicin 45 mg/m^2 I.V. on day 1
Etoposide 100 mg/m^2 I.V. on days 1 through 3
Repeat cycle every 21 days.

Reference: Ardizzoni A, et al. *J Clin Oncol.* 2002;20:3947-3955.

Supportive therapy

Patients are at moderate to high risk for nausea and vomiting, anemia, neutropenia, and diarrhea. Supportive and/or prophylactic therapies are recommended.

Carboplatin, etoposide

Carboplatin to AUC of 5 or 6 I.V. on day 1
Etoposide 100 mg/m^2 I.V. on days 1 through 3
Repeat cycle every 21 to 28 days.

Reference: Pazdur R, et al., eds. *Cancer Management. A Multidisciplinary Approach.* 9th ed. Lawrence, KS: CMP Media; 2005; Skarlos DV, et al. *Ann Oncol.* 2001;12:1231-1238.

Supportive therapy

Patients are at moderate to high risk for nausea and vomiting, anemia, neutropenia, diarrhea, and constipation. Supportive and/or prophylactic therapies are recommended.

Carboplatin, paclitaxel, etoposide

Carboplatin to AUC of 5 or 6 I.V. on day 1
Paclitaxel 135 to 200 mg/m^2 I.V. over 1 hour on day 1
Etoposide 50 mg P.O. alternating with 100 mg P.O. on days 1 through 10
Repeat cycle every 21 days.

Reference: Hainsworth JD, et al. *J Clin Oncol.* 1997;15:3464-3470.

Supportive therapy

Patients are at moderate to high risk for nausea and vomiting, anemia, neutropenia, and hypersensitivity reactions. Supportive and/or prophylactic therapies are recommended.

CAV (cyclophosphamide, doxorubicin [Adriamycin], vincristine)

Cyclophosphamide 800 to 1,000 mg/m^2 I.V. on day 1
Doxorubicin 40 to 50 mg/m^2 I.V. on day 1
Vincristine 1 to 1.4 mg/m^2 I.V. on day 1
Repeat cycle every 21 days.

Reference: Fukuda M, et al. *J Natl Cancer Inst.* 1991;83:855-861; *Facts and Comparisons.* St. Louis, MO: Wolters Kluwer Business; 2005.

See appendices for supportive therapies.

Supportive therapy

Patients are at moderate to high risk for nausea and vomiting, anemia, neutropenia, diarrhea, and constipation. Supportive and/or prophylactic therapies are recommended.

CAV (cyclophosphamide, doxorubicin [Adriamycin], vincristine) alternating with EP (etoposide, cisplatin [Platinol-AQ])

CAV

Cyclophosphamide 1,000 mg/m^2 I.V. on day 1
Doxorubicin 50 mg/m^2 I.V. on day 1
Vincristine 1.2 mg/m^2 I.V. on day 1

EP

Etoposide 100 mg/m^2 I.V. on days 1 through 3
Cisplatin 25 mg/m^2 I.V. on days 1 through 3
Alternate CAV and EP regimens every 21 days.

Reference: Murray N, et al. *J Clin Oncol.* 1999;17:2300-2308.

Supportive therapy

Patients are at moderate to high risk for nausea and vomiting, anemia, neutropenia, diarrhea, constipation, and cisplatin-induced nephrotoxicity. Supportive and/or prophylactic therapies are recommended.

Cisplatin, etoposide

Cisplatin 60 to 80 mg/m^2 I.V. on day 1
Etoposide 80 to 120 mg/m^2 I.V. on days 1 through 3
Repeat cycle every 21 to 28 days.
Or
Cisplatin 25 mg/m^2 I.V. on days 1 through 3
Etoposide 100 mg/m^2 I.V. on days 1 through 3
Repeat cycle every 21 days.

Reference: Pazdur R, et al., eds. *Cancer Management. A Multidisciplinary Approach.* 9th ed. Lawrence, KS: CMP Media; 2005; Turrisi AT 3rd, et al. *N Engl J Med.* 1999;340:265-271; Sundstrom S, et al. *J Clin Oncol.* 2002;20:4665-4672.

Supportive therapy

Patients are at moderate to high risk for nausea and vomiting, anemia, neutropenia, diarrhea, and cisplatin-induced nephrotoxicity. Supportive and/or prophylactic therapies are recommended.

Irinotecan, cisplatin

Cisplatin 60 mg/m² I.V. on day 1
Irinotecan 60 mg/m² I.V. on days 1, 8, and 15
Repeat cycle every 28 days.

Reference: Noda K, et al. *N Engl J Med.* 2002;346:85-91; Pazdur R, et al., eds. *Cancer Management. A Multidisciplinary Approach.* 9th ed. Lawrence, KS: CMP Media; 2005.

Supportive therapy

Patients are at moderate to high risk for nausea and vomiting, anemia, neutropenia, diarrhea, and cisplatin-induced nephrotoxicity. Supportive and/or prophylactic therapies are recommended.

Topotecan

Topotecan 1.5 mg/m² I.V. daily over 30 minutes on days 1 through 5
Repeat every 21 days.

Reference: Schiller JH. *J Clin Oncol.* 2001;19:2114-2122.

Supportive therapy

Patients are at moderate to high risk for nausea and vomiting, anemia, neutropenia, diarrhea, and constipation. Supportive and/or prophylactic therapies are recommended.

Multiple myeloma

Bortezomib

Bortezomib 1.3 mg/m² I.V. on days 1, 4, 8, and 11
Repeat every 21 days.

Reference: Richardson PG, et al. *N Engl J Med.* 2003;348:2609-2617.

Supportive therapy

Patients are at moderate to high risk for nausea and vomiting, anemia, and diarrhea. Supportive and/or prophylactic therapies are recommended.

DVd (pegylated liposomal doxorubicin, vincristine, dexamethasone)

Pegylated liposomal doxorubicin 40 mg/m^2 I.V. on day 1
Vincristine 2 mg I.V. on day 1
Dexamethasone 40 mg P.O. or I.V. on days 1 through 4
Repeat cycle every 28 days for minimum of six cycles and for two cycles after maximum response.

Reference: Hussein MA, et al. *Cancer.* 2002;95:2160-2168.

Supportive therapy

Patients are at moderate to high risk for nausea and vomiting, anemia, and constipation. Supportive and/or prophylactic therapies are recommended.

MP (melphalan, prednisone)

Melphalan 8 to 10 mg/m^2 P.O. on days 1 through 4
Prednisone 60 mg/m^2 P.O. on days 1 through 4
Repeat cycle every 6 weeks.

Reference: Oken MM, et al. *Arch Int Med.* 1975;135:147-152; Oken MM, et al. *Cancer.* 1997;79:1561-1567.

Supportive therapy

Patients are at moderate to high risk for nausea and vomiting, anemia, and neutropenia. Supportive and/or prophylactic therapies are recommended.

Thalidomide, dexamethasone

Thalidomide 200 mg P.O. daily at bedtime for 2 weeks, then increase by 200 mg daily every 2 weeks to maximum of 800 mg daily, as tolerated
Dexamethasone 40 mg P.O. on days 1 through 4, 9 through 12, and 17 through 20 of odd cycles and 40 mg P.O. on days 1 through 4 only during even cycles

Repeat cycle every 28 days.

Reference: Rajkumar SV, et al. *J Clin Oncol.* 2002;20:4319-4323.

Supportive therapy

Patients are at moderate to high risk for nausea and vomiting, anemia, and deep vein thrombosis. Supportive and/or prophylactic therapies are recommended.

VAD (vincristine, doxorubicin [Adriamycin], dexamethasone)

Vincristine 0.4 mg daily by continuous I.V. infusion on days 1 through 4
Doxorubicin 9 mg/m^2 daily by continuous I.V. infusion on days 1 through 4
Dexamethasone 40 mg P.O.on days 1 through 4, 9 through 12, and 17 through 20

Repeat cycle every 28 days.

Reference: Barlogie B, et al. *N Engl J Med.* 1984;310:1353-1356; Alexian R. *Am J Hematol.* 1990;33:86-89.

Supportive therapy

Patients are at moderate to high risk for nausea and vomiting, anemia, neutropenia, and constipation. Supportive and/or prophylactic therapies are recommended.

Myelodysplastic syndrome

Azacitidine

Azacitidine 75 mg/m^2 subcutaneously daily for 7 days
Repeat every 28 days.

Reference: Silverman LR, et al. *J Clin Oncol.* 2002;20:2429-2440.

Supportive therapy

Patients are at moderate to high risk for nausea and vomiting, anemia, and neutropenia. Supportive and/or prophylactic therapies are recommended.

Neuroendocrine tumors

Doxorubicin, streptozocin

Streptozocin 500 mg/m^2 I.V. on days 1 through 5
Doxorubicin 50 mg/m^2 I.V. on days 1 and 22
Repeat cycle every 6 weeks.

Reference: Moertel CG, et al. *N Engl J Med.* 1992;326:519.

Supportive therapy

Patients are at moderate to high risk for nausea and vomiting, anemia, and neutropenia. Supportive and/or prophylactic therapies are recommended.

Non-Hodgkin's lymphoma

Chlorambucil

Chlorambucil 40 mg/m^2 P.O. on day 1
Repeat every 28 days.

Reference: Rai KR, et al. *N Engl J Med.* 2000;343:1750-1757.

Supportive therapy

Patients are at moderate to high risk for nausea and vomiting, anemia, neutropenia, and diarrhea. Supportive and/or prophylactic therapies are recommended.

CHOP (cyclophosphamide, doxorubicin, vincristine [Oncovin], prednisone)

Cyclophosphamide 750 mg/m^2 I.V. on day 1
Doxorubicin 50 mg/m^2 I.V. on day 1
Vincristine 1.4 mg/m^2 I.V. on day 1
Prednisone 100 mg P.O. on days 1 through 5
Repeat cycle every 21 days.

Reference: Doorduijin JK, et al. *J Clin Oncol.* 2003;21:3041-3050.

Supportive therapy

Patients are at moderate to high risk for nausea and vomiting, anemia,

neutropenia, diarrhea, and constipation. Supportive and/or prophylactic therapies are recommended.

CODOX-M (cyclophosphamide, vincristine [Oncovin], doxorubicin, high-dose methotrexate) alternating with IVAC (ifosfamide, etoposide, high-dose cytarabine)

CODOX-M

Cyclophosphamide 800 mg/m^2 I.V. on day 1 *and* 200 mg/m^2 I.V. on days 2 through 5

Vincristine 1.5 mg/m^2 I.V. on days 1 and 8 in cycle 1 and days 1, 8, and 15 in cycle 3

Doxorubicin 40 mg/m^2 I.V. on day 1

Cytarabine 70 mg intrathecally on days 1 and 3

Methotrexate 1,200 mg/m^2 I.V. over 1 hour on day 1 followed by 240 mg/m^2 every hour for 23 hours on day 10

Leucovorin 192 mg/m^2 I.V. begun 12 hours after completion of methotrexate for one dose, followed by 12 mg/m^2 I.V. every 6 hours until methotrexate level is below 5×10^{-8} mol/L

Methotrexate 12 mg intrathecally on day 15

Patients presenting with CNS disease receive additional intrathecal therapy with cytarabine on day 5 and methotrexate on day 17.

IVAC

Etoposide 60 mg/m^2 I.V. over 1 hour on days 1 through 5

Ifosfamide 1,500 mg/m^2 I.V. over 1 hour on days 1 through 5 with mesna 360 mg/m^2 I.V., followed by 360 mg/m^2 I.V. every 3 hours over 15 minutes on days 1 through 5

Cytarabine 2,000 mg/m^2 I.V. over 3 hours every 12 hours on days 1 and 2 (four doses total)

Methotrexate 12 mg intrathecally on day 5

Leucovorin 15 mg P.O. 24 hours after intrathecal methotrexate

Patients presenting with CNS disease receive additional intrathecal therapy with cytarabine 70 mg on days 7 and 9 of first IVAC regimen.

Alternate CODOX-M and IVAC regimens for total of four cycles (two of each).

Reference: Magrath I, et al. *J Clin Oncol.* 1996;14:925-934; Mead GM, et al. *Annals Oncol.* 2002;13:1264-1274.

Supportive therapy

Patients are at moderate to high risk for nausea and vomiting, anemia, and neutropenia. Supportive and/or prophylactic therapies are recommended.

Fludarabine, rituximab

Fludarabine 25 mg/m^2 I.V. on days 1 through 5
Rituximab 375 mg/m^2 I.V. on days 1, 8, 15, and 22
Repeat cycle every 21 to 28 days.
Reference: Czuczman MS, et al. *J Clin Oncol.* 2005;23:694-704.

Supportive therapy

Patients are at moderate to high risk for nausea and vomiting, anemia, and constipation. Supportive and/or prophylactic therapies are recommended.

Hyper CVAD (cyclophosphamide, vincristine, doxorubicin [Adriamycin], dexamethasone) alternating with methotrexate, cytarabine

Hyper CVAD

Cyclophosphamide 300 mg/m^2 I.V. over 3 hours every 12 hours (for six doses) on days 1 through 3 and mesna at same total dose of cyclophosphamide by continuous I.V. infusion, starting with the first cyclophosphamide dose and ending 6 hours after last dose
Vincristine 2 mg I.V. on days 4 and 11
Dexamethasone 40 mg daily I.V. or P.O. on days 1 through 4 and days 11 through 14
Doxorubicin 50 mg/m^2 I.V. on day 4

Methotrexate, cytarabine

Methotrexate 200 mg/^{2} I.V. over 2 hours on day 1, then 800 mg/m^2 I.V. over 24 hours
Cytarabine 3,000 mg/m^2 I.V. over 2 hours every 12 hours for four doses on days 2 and 3
Methylprednisolone 50 mg I.V. twice daily (for six doses) on days 1 through 3
Leucovorin 15 mg I.V. or P.O. every 6 hours until methotrexate level is below 5×10^{-8} mol/L starting 24 hours after methotrexate

Alternate both regimens for total of eight cycles (four of each).

Reference: Kantarjian HM, et al. *J Clin Oncol.* 2000;18:547-561.

Supportive therapy

Patients are at moderate to high risk for nausea and vomiting, anemia, neutropenia, diarrhea, CNS disease, hyperuricemia, conjunctivitis, infection, and methotrexate-induced nephrotoxicity. Supportive and/or prophylactic therapies are recommended.

Rituximab

Rituximab 375 mg/m^2 by slow I.V. infusion once weekly for four or eight doses

Reference: Witzig TE, et al. *J Clin Oncol.* 2005;23:1103-1108.

Supportive therapy

Patients are at moderate to high risk for nausea and vomiting, anemia, and infusion reactions. Supportive and/or prophylactic therapies are recommended.

Rituximab/CHOP (cyclophosphamide, doxorubicin, vincristine [Oncovin], prednisone)

Rituximab 375 mg/m^2 I.V. on day 1
Cyclophosphamide 750 mg/m^2 I.V. on day 1
Doxorubicin 50 mg/m^2 I.V. on day 1
Vincristine 1.4 mg/m^2 I.V. on day 1
Prednisone 100 mg P.O. on days 1 through 5
Repeat cycle every 21 days.

Reference: Zinzani PL, et al. *J Clin Oncol.* 2004;22:2654-2661.

Supportive therapy

Patients are at moderate to high risk for nausea and vomiting, anemia, neutropenia, diarrhea, constipation, and infusion reactions. Supportive and/or prophylactic therapies are recommended.

Rituximab/EPOCH (etoposide, prednisone, vincristine [Oncovin], doxorubicin, cyclophosphamide)

Rituximab 375 mg/m^2 I.V. on day 1
Etoposide 50 mg/m^2 daily (by continuous I.V. infusion over 96 hours) on days 1 through 4

Vincristine 0.4 mg/m^2 daily (by continuous I.V. infusion over 96 hours) on days 1 through 4

Doxorubicin 10 mg/m^2 by daily (continuous I.V. infusion over 96 hours) on days 1 through 4

Prednisone 60 mg/m^2 P.O. on days 1 through 5

Cyclophosphamide 750 mg/m^2 I.V. on day 5

Repeat cycle every 21 days.

Reference: Gutierrez M, et al. *J Clin Oncol.* 2000;18:3633-3642; Pazdur R, et al., eds. *Cancer Management. A Multidisciplinary Approach.* 9th ed. Lawrence, KS: CMP Media; 2005.

Supportive therapy

Patients are at moderate to high risk for nausea and vomiting, anemia, neutropenia, diarrhea, constipation, and infusion reactions. Supportive and/or prophylactic therapies are recommended.

Rituximab/hyper CVAD (cyclophosphamide, vincristine, doxorubicin [Adriamycin], dexamethasone) alternating with methotrexate, cytarabine

Rituximab/hyper CVAD

Rituximab 375 mg/m^2 I.V. on day 1

Cyclophosphamide 300 mg/m^2 I.V. every 12 hours on days 2 through 4 infused over 3 hours for total of six doses

Doxorubicin 16.7 mg/m^2 I.V. daily over 24 hours on days 5 through 7

Vincristine 1.4 mg/m^2 I.V. on days 5 and 12

Dexamethasone 40 mg I.V. or P.O.daily on days 2 through 5 and days 12 through 15

Methotrexate, cytarabine

Rituximab 375 mg/m^2 I.V. on day 1

Methotrexate 200 mg/m^2 I.V. over 2 hours, then 800 mg/m^2 by continuous I.V. infusion over 22 hours on day 2

Cytarabine 3,000 mg/m^2 I.V. (over 2 hours) every 12 hours for four doses on days 3 through 4

Leucovorin 15 mg P.O. or I.V. every 6 hours until methotrexate level is below 5×10^{-8} mol/L, starting after methotrexate

Alternate regimens every 21 days for total of six to eight cycles.

Reference: Romaguera JE. *J Clin Oncol.* 2005;23:7013-7023.

Supportive therapy

Patients are at moderate to high risk for nausea and vomiting, anemia, neutropenia, diarrhea, and infusion reactions. Supportive and/or prophylactic therapies are recommended.

Ovarian cancer

Carboplatin, cyclophosphamide

Carboplatin 300 mg/m^2 I.V. on day 1
Cyclophosphamide 600 mg/m^2 I.V. on day 1
Repeat cycle every 28 days for six cycles.

Reference: Alberts DS, et al. *J Clin Oncol.* 1992;10:706-717; Swenerton K, et al. *J Clin Oncol.* 1992;10:718-726.

Supportive therapy

Patients are at moderate to high risk for nausea and vomiting, anemia, neutropenia, diarrhea, and constipation. Supportive and/or prophylactic therapies are recommended.

Cisplatin, etoposide

Cisplatin 50 to 70 mg/m^2 I.V. weekly for 6 weeks
Etoposide 50 mg P.O. once daily for 6 weeks

Reference: van der Burg ME, et al. *Br J Cancer.* 2002;86:19-25.

Supportive therapy

Patients are at moderate to high risk for nausea and vomiting, anemia, neutropenia, diarrhea, and cisplatin-induced nephrotoxicity. Supportive and/or prophylactic therapies are recommended.

Docetaxel, carboplatin

Docetaxel 60 mg/m^2 I.V. on day 1, followed by
Carboplatin to AUC of 6 I.V.
Repeat cycle every 21 days.

Reference: Markman M, et al. *J Clin Oncol.* 2001;19:1901-1905.

Supportive therapy

Patients are at moderate to high risk for nausea and vomiting, anemia,

neutropenia, diarrhea, constipation, and hypersensitivity reactions. Supportive and/or prophylactic therapies are recommended.

Paclitaxel

Paclitaxel 175 mg/m^2 I.V. over 3 hours on day 1
Repeat every 21 days.

Reference: Eisenhauer EA, et al. *J Clin Oncol.* 1994;12:2654-2666; Markman M, et al. *J Clin Oncol.* 2003;21:2460-2465.

Supportive therapy
Patients are at moderate to high risk for nausea and vomiting, anemia, neutropenia, and hypersensitivity reactions. Supportive and/or prophylactic therapies are recommended.

Paclitaxel, carboplatin

Paclitaxel 175 mg/m^2 I.V. over 3 hours on day 1, followed by
Carboplatin to AUC of 5 to 7.5 I.V. over 1 hour on day 1
Repeat cycle every 21 days.

Reference: Vasey PA, et al. *J Natl Cancer Inst.* 2004;96:1682-1691; Coleman RL, et al. *Cancer J Sci Am.* 1997;3:246-253.

Supportive therapy
Patients are at moderate to high risk for nausea and vomiting, anemia, neutropenia, diarrhea, constipation, and hypersensitivity reactions. Supportive and/or prophylactic therapies are recommended.

Paclitaxel, cisplatin

Paclitaxel 135 mg/m^2 I.V. over 3 hours on day 1, followed by
Cisplatin 75 mg/m^2 I.V. over 1 hour on day 1
Repeat cycle every 21 days.

Reference: McGuire WP, et al. *N Engl J Med.* 1996;334:1-6; Neijt JP, et al. *J Clin Oncol.* 2000;18:3084-3092; Ozols RF, et al. *J Clin Oncol.* 2003;21:3194-3200.

Supportive therapy
Patients are at moderate to high risk for nausea and vomiting, anemia, neutropenia, diarrhea, hypersensitivity reactions, and cisplatin-induced nephrotoxicity. Supportive and/or prophylactic therapies are recommended.

Pancreatic cancer

Capecitabine

Capecitabine 1,250 mg/m^2 P.O. twice daily on days 1 through 14
Repeat every 21 days.

Reference: Cartwright TH, et al. *J Clin Oncol.* 2002;20:160-164.

Supportive therapy
Patients are at moderate to high risk for nausea and vomiting, anemia, and diarrhea. Supportive and/or prophylactic therapies are recommended.

Gemcitabine

Gemcitabine 1,000 mg/m^2 I.V. every week for 7 weeks, followed by 1 week of rest
Repeat subsequent cycles 3 weeks out of every 4.

Reference: Costanzo FD, et al. *Br J Cancer.* 2005;93:185-189.

Supportive therapy
Patients are at moderate to high risk for nausea and vomiting, anemia, and neutropenia. Supportive and/or prophylactic therapies are recommended.

Gemcitabine, cisplatin

Gemcitabine 1,000 mg/m^2 I.V. over 30 minutes on days 1, 8, and 15, followed by
Cisplatin 50 mg/m^2 I.V. on days 1 and 15
Repeat cycle every 28 days.

Reference: Philip PA, et al. *Cancer.* 2001;92:569-577.

Supportive therapy
Patients are at moderate to high risk for nausea and vomiting, anemia, neutropenia, diarrhea, and cisplatin-induced nephrotoxicity. Supportive and/or prophylactic therapies are recommended.

Gemcitabine, oxaliplatin

Gemcitabine 1,000 mg/m^2 I.V. over 100 minutes (10 mg/m^2/minute) on day 1

Oxaliplatin 100 mg/m^2 I.V. over 2 hours on day 2

Repeat cycle every 14 days.

Reference: Louvet C, et al. *J Clin Oncol.* 2002;20:1512-1518.

Supportive therapy

Patients are at moderate to high risk for nausea and vomiting and anemia. Supportive and/or prophylactic therapies are recommended.

Prostate cancer

Docetaxel, estramustine

Estramustine 280 mg P.O. three times daily on days 1 through 5

Docetaxel 60 mg/m^2 I.V. on day 2

Repeat cycle every 21 days for maximum of six cycles.

Reference: Walczak JR, et al. *Urology.* 2003;62(suppl 1):141-146.

Supportive therapy

Patients are at moderate to high risk for nausea and vomiting, neutropenia, and hypersensitivity reactions. Supportive and/or prophylactic therapies are recommended.

Docetaxel, prednisone

Docetaxel 75 mg/m^2 I.V. over 1 hour on day 1

Prednisone 5 mg P.O. twice daily on days 1 through 21

Repeat cycle every 21 days.

Reference: Tannock IF, et al. *N Engl J Med.* 2004;351:1502-1512.

Supportive therapy

Patients are at moderate to high risk for nausea and vomiting, neutropenia, and hypersensitivity reactions. Supportive and/or prophylactic therapies are recommended.

Estramustine, vinblastine

Estramustine 600 mg/m^2 P.O. in divided doses daily on days 1 through 42

Vinblastine 4 mg/m^2 I.V. weekly for 6 weeks, beginning on day 1

Repeat cycle every 8 weeks.

Reference: Hudes G, et al. *J Clin Oncol.* 1999;17:3160-3166.

Supportive therapy

Patients are at moderate to high risk for nausea and vomiting, anemia, and constipation. Supportive and/or prophylactic therapies are recommended.

Hormone therapy

Bicalutamide and leuprolide or goserelin

Bicalutamide 50 mg daily P.O.

Leuprolide depot 7.5 mg I.M. every 28 days

Or

Goserelin implant 3.6 mg subcutaneously every 28 days

Reference: Schellhammer P, et al. *Urology.* 1995;45:745-752.

FL (flutamide and leuprolide)

Flutamide 250 mg P.O. three times daily

Leuprolide 1 mg daily subcutaneously

Or

Leuprolide depot 7.5 mg I.M. every 28 days

Reference: Sarosdy MF, et al. *Urology.* 2000;55:391-396.

FZ (flutamide and goserelin [Zoladex])

Flutamide 250 mg P.O. three times daily

Goserelin implant 3.6 mg subcutaneously every 28 days, beginning 8 weeks before radiation therapy for four cycles; or 10.8 mg subcutaneously 4 weeks before radiotherapy

Reference: Jurincic CD, et al. *Semin Oncol.* 1991;18(suppl 6):21-25.

Goserelin, leuprolide, or triptorelin

Goserelin implant 3.6 mg subcutaneously every 28 days; or 10.8 mg subcutaneously every 12 weeks

Reference: Pilepich MV, et al. *Urology.* 1995;45:616-623.

Or

Leuprolide depot 7.5 mg I.M. every 28 days or 22.5 mg I.M. every 3

---

months; or 30 mg I.M. every 4 months

Reference: Lupron Depot 7.5 mg, Lupron Depot 22.5 mg, Lupron Depot 30 mg [package inserts]. Lake Forest, IL: TAP Pharmaceuticals; 2004. Or

Triptorelin 3.75 mg I.M. every 28 days; or triptorelin LA 11.25 mg I.M. every 84 days

Reference: Kuhn JM, et al. *Eur Urol.* 1997;32:397-403.

Supportive therapy

Patients are at moderate to high risk for nausea and vomiting and osteoporosis. Supportive and/or prophylactic therapies are recommended.

PE (paclitaxel, estramustine)

Paclitaxel 120 mg/m² I.V. daily on days 1 through 4 (continuous infusion over 96 hours)
Estramustine 600 mg/m² P.O. daily in two or three divided doses, starting 24 hours before paclitaxel
Repeat cycle every 21 days.

Reference: Hudes GR, et al. *J Clin Oncol.* 1997;15:3156-3163.

Supportive therapy

Patients are at moderate to high risk for nausea and vomiting, anemia, neutropenia, diarrhea, and hypersensitivity reactions. Supportive and/or prophylactic therapies are recommended.

Skin cancer (melanoma)

Aldesleukin (interleukin-2)

Aldesleukin 600,000 units/kg I.V. over 15 minutes every 8 hours for 5 days for maximum of 14 doses
Repeat after 9 days of rest.

Reference: Atkins MB, et al. *Cancer J Sci Am.* 2000;6(suppl 1):S11–S14.

Supportive therapy

Patients are at moderate to high risk for nausea and vomiting, anemia, and diarrhea. Supportive and/or prophylactic therapies are recommended.

Dacarbazine

Dacarbazine 2 to 4.5 mg/kg I.V. daily on days 1 through 10
Repeat every 21 or 28 days.
Or
Dacarbazine 1,000 mg/m^2 I.V. on day 1
Repeat every 21 days.

Reference: Chapman PB, et al. *J Clin Oncol.* 1999;17:2745-2751; Middleton MR, et al. *J Clin Oncol.* 2000;18:158-166.

Supportive therapy

Patients are at moderate to high risk for nausea and vomiting, anemia, and neutropenia. Supportive and/or prophylactic therapies are recommended.

IFN (interferon alfa-2b)

Interferon alfa-2b 20 million units/m^2 I.V. weekly on days 1 through 5 for 4 weeks, then 10 million units/m^2 subcutaneously three times weekly for 48 weeks

Reference: Kirkwood JM, et al. *J Clin Oncol.* 1996;14:7-17.

Supportive therapy

Patients are at moderate to high risk for nausea and vomiting, neutropenia, and flulike symptoms. Supportive and/or prophylactic therapies are recommended.

Temozolomide

Temozolomide 200 mg/m^2 P.O. on days 1 through 5
Repeat every 28 days.

Reference: Middleton MR, et al. *Am Soc Clin Oncol.* 2000;18:158-166.

Supportive therapy

Patients are at moderate to high risk for nausea and vomiting, neutropenia, and constipation. Supportive and/or prophylactic therapies are recommended.

Skin cancer (Merkel cell)

Carboplatin, etoposide

Carboplatin to AUC of 4.5 I.V. on day 1 of weeks 1, 4, 7, and 10
Etoposide 80 mg/m^2 I.V. daily on days 1 through 3 of weeks 1, 4, 7, and 10

Reference: Poulsen M, et al. *J Clin Oncol.* 2003;21:4371-4376.

Supportive therapy

Patients are at moderate to high risk for nausea and vomiting, anemia, neutropenia, diarrhea, and constipation. Supportive and/or prophylactic therapies are recommended.

Topotecan

Topotecan 1.5 mg/m^2 I.V. over 30 minutes on days 1 through 5
Repeat every 21 days.

Reference: NCCN Practice Guidelines in Oncology. Merkel Cell Carcinoma v.2.2005. Available in: Hycamtin prescribing information. Research Triangle Park, NC: GlaxoSmithKline; July 2003.

Supportive therapy

Patients are at moderate to high risk for nausea and vomiting, anemia, neutropenia, diarrhea, and constipation. Supportive and/or prophylactic therapies are recommended.

Soft-tissue sarcoma

AD (doxorubicin [Adriamycin], dacarbazine)

Doxorubicin 15 mg/m^2 daily by continuous I.V. infusion on days 1 through 4
Dacarbazine 250 mg/m^2 daily by continuous I.V. infusion on days 1 through 4
Repeat cycle every 21 days.

Reference: Antman K, et al. *J Clin Oncol.* 1993;11:1276-1285.

Supportive therapy

Patients are at moderate to high risk for nausea and vomiting, anemia,

and neutropenia. Supportive and/or prophylactic therapies are recommended.

AIM (doxorubicin [Adriamycin], ifosfamide, mesna)

Doxorubicin 50 mg/m^2 by I.V. bolus on day 1
Ifosfamide 5,000 mg/m^2 by continuous I.V. infusion on day 1
Mesna 600 mg/m^2 by I.V. bolus before ifosfamide, 2,500 mg/m^2 by continuous I.V. infusion with ifosfamide, and 1,250 mg/m^2 I.V. over 12 hours following ifosfamide
Repeat cycle every 21 days.

Reference: Santoro A, et al. *J Clin Oncol.* 1995;13:1537-1545.

Supportive therapy
Patients are at moderate to high risk for nausea and vomiting, anemia, and neutropenia. Supportive and/or prophylactic therapies are recommended.

Doxorubicin

Doxorubicin 75 mg/m^2 I.V. on day 1
Repeat every 21 days.

Reference: Edmonson JH, et al. *J Clin Oncol.* 1993;11:1269-1275; Nielsen OS, et al. *Br J Cancer.* 1998;78:1634-1639; Santoro A, et al. *J Clin Oncol.* 1995;13:1537-1545.

Supportive therapy
Patients are at moderate to high risk for nausea and vomiting, anemia, and neutropenia. Supportive and/or prophylactic therapies are recommended.

Gemcitabine, docetaxel

For patients who have previously received radiation:
Gemcitabine 675 mg/m^2 I.V. over 90 minutes on days 1 and 8
Docetaxel 100 mg/m^2 I.V. over 60 minutes on day 8
Repeat cycle every 21 days.
Or
For patients who have not previously received radiation:
Gemcitabine 900 mg/m^2 I.V. over 90 minutes on days 1 and 8
Docetaxel 100 mg/m^2 I.V. over 60 minutes on day 8

See appendices for supportive therapies.

Repeat cycle every 21 days.

Reference: Leu KM, et al. *J Clin Oncol.* 2004;22:1706-1712; Hensley ML. *J Clin Oncol.* 2002;20:2824-2831.

Supportive therapy

Patients are at moderate to high risk for nausea and vomiting, anemia, neutropenia, diarrhea, and hypersensitivity reactions. Supportive and/or prophylactic therapies are recommended.

Imatinib mesylate

Imatinib mesylate 400 to 800 mg P.O. daily for 8 weeks or more as tolerated

Reference: Demetri GD, et al. *N Engl J Med.* 2002;347:472-480; Verweij J, et al. *Lancet.* 2004;364:1127-1134.

Supportive therapy

Patients are at moderate to high risk for nausea and vomiting, anemia, and neutropenia. Supportive and/or prophylactic therapies are recommended.

MAID (mesna, doxorubicin [Adriamycin], ifosfamide, dacarbazine)

Regimen A

Ifosfamide 2,500 mg/m^2 daily by continuous I.V. infusion on days 1 through 3

Mesna 2,500 mg/m^2 daily by continuous I.V. infusion on days 1 through 4

Doxorubicin 15 mg/m^2 daily by continuous I.V. infusion on days 1 through 4

Dacarbazine 250 mg/m^2 daily by continuous I.V. infusion on days 1 through 4

Repeat cycle every 21 days.

Reference: Antman K, et al. *J Clin Oncol.* 1993;11:1276-1285.

Or

Regimen B

Ifosfamide 2,500 mg/m^2 daily by continuous I.V. infusion on days 1 through 3

Mesna 2,500 mg/m^2 daily by continuous I.V. infusion on days 1 through 4

Doxorubicin 20 mg/m^2 daily by continuous I.V. infusion on days 1 through 3

Dacarbazine 300 mg/m^2 daily by continuous I.V. infusion on days 1 through 3

Repeat cycle every 21 days.

Reference: Elias A, et al. *Semin Oncol.* 1990;17(suppl 4):41-49.

Supportive therapy

Patients are at moderate to high risk for nausea and vomiting, anemia, and neutropenia. Supportive and/or prophylactic therapies are recommended.

Testicular cancer

BEP (bleomycin, etoposide, cisplatin [Platinol-AQ])

Etoposide 100 mg/m^2 I.V. daily over 30 to 60 minutes on days 1 through 5

Cisplatin 20 mg/m^2 I.V. over 30 to 60 minutes on days 1 through 5

Bleomycin 30 units by I.V. bolus on days 2, 9, and 16

Repeat cycle every 21 days.

Reference: Williams SD, et al. *N Engl J Med.* 1987;316:1435-1440.

Supportive therapy

Patients are at moderate to high risk for nausea and vomiting, anemia, neutropenia, and cisplatin-induced nephrotoxicity. Supportive and/or prophylactic therapies are recommended.

EP (etoposide, cisplatin [Platinol-AQ])

Etoposide 100 mg/m^2 I.V. daily on days 1 through 5

Cisplatin 20 mg/m^2 I.V. daily on days 1 through 5

Repeat cycle once after 21 days.

Reference: Motzer RJ, et al. *J Clin Oncol.* 1995;13:2700-2704.

Supportive therapy

Patients are at moderate to high risk for nausea and vomiting, anemia,

neutropenia, and cisplatin-induced nephrotoxicity. Supportive and/or prophylactic therapies are recommended.

Paclitaxel, ifosfamide, cisplatin, mesna

Paclitaxel 250 mg/m^2 by continuous I.V. infusion over 24 hours on day 1
Ifosfamide 1,500 mg/m^2 by I.V. infusion over 60 minutes on days 2 through 5 given with *Mesna* 500 mg/m^2 I.V. before ifosfamide and 4 and 8 hours after ifosfamide for total daily mesna dose of 1,500 mg/m^2 to match daily ifosfamide dose on days 2 through 5
Cisplatin 25 mg/m^2 by I.V. infusion over 30 minutes on days 2 through 5
Repeat cycle every 21 days.

Reference: Kondagunta GV, et al. *J Clin Oncol.* 2005;23:6549-6555; Motzer RJ, et al. *J Clin Oncol.* 2000;18:2413-2418.

Supportive therapy
Patients are at moderate to high risk for nausea and vomiting, anemia, neutropenia, diarrhea, hypersensitivity reactions, and cisplatin-induced nephrotoxicity. Supportive and/or prophylactic therapies are recommended.

PVB (cisplatin [Platinol-AQ], vinblastine, bleomycin)

Vinblastine 0.15 mg/kg daily by I.V. bolus on days 1 and 2
Cisplatin 20 mg/m^2 I.V. daily over 15 to 30 minutes on days 1 through 5
Bleomycin 30 units daily by I.V. bolus on days 2, 9, and 16
Repeat cycle every 21 days.

Reference: Williams SD, et al. *N Engl J Med.* 1987;316:1435-1440.

Supportive therapy
Patients are at moderate to high risk for nausea and vomiting, anemia, neutropenia, constipation, and cisplatin-induced nephrotoxicity. Supportive and/or prophylactic therapies are recommended.

VelP (vinblastine, ifosfamide, mesna, cisplatin [Platinol-AQ])

Vinblastine 0.11 mg/kg I.V. daily on days 1 and 2
Ifosfamide 1,200 mg/m^2 daily on days 1 through 5 by continuous I.V. infusion with *mesna* 400 mg I.V. daily 15 minutes before ifosfamide, followed by 1,200 mg continuous I.V. infusion daily on days 1 through 5

Cisplatin 20 mg/m^2 I.V. over 30 to 60 minutes on days 1 through 5
Repeat cycle every 21 days.

Reference: Loehrer PJ, et al. *Ann Intern Med.* 1988;109:540-546.

Supportive therapy
Patients are at moderate to high risk for nausea and vomiting, anemia, neutropenia, constipation, and cisplatin-induced nephrotoxicity. Supportive and/or prophylactic therapies are recommended.

VIP (etoposide [VePesid], ifosfamide, mesna, cisplatin [Platinol-AQ])

Etoposide 75 mg/m^2 I.V. daily on days 1 through 5
Ifosfamide 1,200 mg/m^2 I.V. daily on days 1 through 5 given with *mesna* 400 mg I.V. 15 minutes before ifosfamide, followed by 1,200 mg daily by continuous I.V. infusion on days 1 through 5
Cisplatin 20 mg/m^2 I.V. over 30 to 60 minutes on days 1 through 5
Repeat cycle every 21 days.

Reference: Loehrer PJ, et al. *Ann Intern Med.* 1988;109:540-546.

Supportive therapy
Patients are at moderate to high risk for nausea and vomiting, anemia, neutropenia, and cisplatin-induced nephrotoxicity. Supportive and/or prophylactic therapies are recommended.

Thyroid cancer

CVD (cyclophosphamide, vincristine, dacarbazine)

Cyclophosphamide 750 mg/m^2 I.V. on day 1
Vincristine 1.4 mg/m^2 I.V. on day 1
Dacarbazine 600 mg/m^2 I.V. on days 1 and 2
Repeat cycle every 21 to 28 days.

Reference: Wu LT, et al. *Cancer.* 1994;73:432-436.

Supportive therapy
Patients are at moderate to high risk for nausea and vomiting, anemia, neutropenia, and diarrhea. Supportive and/or prophylactic therapies are recommended.

Uterine cancer

CAP (cyclophosphamide, doxorubicin [Adriamycin], cisplatin [Platinol-AQ])

Cisplatin 70 mg/m^2 I.V. on day 1
Doxorubicin 40 mg/m^2 I.V. on day 1
Cyclophosphamide 500 mg/m^2 I.V. on day 1
Repeat cycle every 28 days.

Reference: Watanabe Y, et al. *Gynecol Oncol.* 2004;94:333-339.

Supportive therapy
Patients are at moderate to high risk for nausea and vomiting, anemia, neutropenia, diarrhea, and cisplatin-induced nephrotoxicity. Supportive and/or prophylactic therapies are recommended.

Cisplatin, doxorubicin

Cisplatin 100 mg/m^2 I.V. on day 1
Doxorubicin 45 to 60 mg/m^2 I.V. on day 1
Repeat cycle every 21 days.

Reference: Peters WA III, et al. *Gynecol Oncol.* 1989;34:323-327; Randall ME, et al. *J Clin Oncol.* 2003;22:237.

Supportive therapy
Patients are at moderate to high risk for nausea and vomiting, anemia, neutropenia, diarrhea, and cisplatin-induced nephrotoxicity. Supportive and/or prophylactic therapies are recommended.

Cisplatin, paclitaxel

Radiation therapy, days 1 and 28: 4,500 cGy in 5 weeks, with daily fractions of 1.8 Gy to pelvis, followed by intracavitary single low dose of 20 Gy to vaginal surface; or three high-dose applications totaling 18 Gy to vaginal surface
Cisplatin 50 mg/m^2 I.V. on days 1 and 28
After radiation therapy is completed:
Cisplatin 50 mg/m^2 I.V. on day 1
Paclitaxel 175 mg/m^2 I.V. over 24 hours on day 1

Repeat cisplatin and paclitaxel every 28 days.

Reference: Greven K, et al. *Int J Radiat Oncol Biol Phys.* 2004;59:168-173.

Supportive therapy

Patients are at moderate to high risk for nausea and vomiting, anemia, neutropenia, diarrhea, hypersensitivity reactions, and cisplatin-induced nephrotoxicity. Supportive and/or prophylactic therapies are recommended.

Doxorubicin

Doxorubicin 60 mg/m^2 I.V. on day 1
Repeat every 28 days.

Reference: Thigpen JT, et al. *J Clin Oncol.* 2004;22:3902-3908; Aapro MS, et al. *Ann Oncol.* 2003;14:441-448.

Supportive therapy

Patients are at moderate to high risk for nausea and vomiting and neutropenia. Supportive and/or prophylactic therapies are recommended.

Ifosfamide, cisplatin

Ifosfamide 1,500 mg/m^2 I.V. daily given with mesna 1,500 mg/m^2 daily by continuous I.V. infusion on days 1 through 5
Cisplatin 20 mg/m^2 I.V. daily on days 1 through 5
Repeat cycle every 21 days.

Reference: Sutton G, et al. *Gynecol Oncol.* 2000;79:147-153.

Supportive therapy

Patients are at moderate to high risk for nausea and vomiting, anemia, neutropenia, and cisplatin-induced nephrotoxicity. Supportive and/or prophylactic therapies are recommended.

MAID (mesna, doxorubicin [Adriamycin], ifosfamide, dacarbazine)

Ifosfamide 2,500 mg/m^2 daily by continuous I.V. infusion on days 1 through 3
Mesna 2,500 mg/m^2 daily by continuous I.V. infusion on days 1 through 4
Doxorubicin 15 mg/m^2 daily by continuous I.V. infusion on days 1 through 4

See appendices for supportive therapies.

Dacarbazine 250 mg/m^2 daily by continuous I.V. infusion on days 1 through 4

Repeat cycle every 21 days.

Reference: Antman K, et al. *J Clin Oncol.* 1993;11:1276-1285.

Supportive therapy

Patients are at moderate to high risk for nausea and vomiting, anemia, and neutropenia. Supportive and/or prophylactic therapies are recommended.

TAP (doxorubicin [Adriamycin], cisplatin [Platinol-AQ], paclitaxel [Taxol], filgrastim)

Doxorubicin 45 mg/m^2 I.V. on day 1, followed immediately by
Cisplatin 50 mg/m^2 I.V. on day 1
Paclitaxel 160 mg/m^2 I.V. over 3 hours on day 2
Filgrastim 5 mcg/kg subcutaneously on days 3 through 12

Repeat cycle every 21 days for maximum of seven cycles.

Reference: Fleming GF, et al. *J Clin Oncol.* 2004;22:2159-2166.

Supportive therapy

Patients are at moderate to high risk for nausea and vomiting, anemia, neutropenia, diarrhea, hypersensitivity reactions, and cisplatin-induced nephrotoxicity. Supportive and/or prophylactic therapies are recommended.

Common oncology abbreviations

The abbreviations below are commonly used in oncology practice and research. However, use abbreviations with caution. When in doubt, spell out the word or term rather than risk misinterpretation of an abbreviation.

AA	anaplastic anemia
AAIR	age-adjusted incidence rate
ABMT	autologous bone marrow transplant
ADE	adverse drug event
ADR	adverse drug reaction
AE	adverse event
AFP	alpha fetoprotein
ALCL	anaplastic large-cell lymphoma
ALL	acute lymphoblastic or lymphocytic leukemia
AML	acute myeloid leukemia
ANA	antinuclear antibodies
ANC	absolute neutrophil count
ANLL	acute nonlymphocytic leukemia
Ara-C	cytarabine
AUC	area under the curve
BCL	B-cell leukemia, B-cell lymphoma
BCNU	carmustine
bleo	bleomycin
BMT	bone marrow transplant
BRM	biological response modifier
BSA	body surface area
BSE	breast self-examination
Bx	biopsy
CA	cancer, cancer antigen
CA 125	cancer antigen 125
CCNU	lomustine
CEA	carcinoembryonic antigen
CG	control group
CGL	chronic granulocytic leukemia
cGy	centigray (unit of radiation)
CIS	carcinoma in situ
CR	complete remission, complete response
CRA	clinical research associate
CSF	colony-stimulating factor, cerebrospinal fluid
CT	computerized tomography
CTC	common toxicity criteria (research and clinical tool to assess toxicity)
CTCL	cutaneous T-cell lymphoma
DCIS	ductal carcinoma in situ

DFI	disease-free interval	HPV	human papillomavirus
DLBCL	diffuse large B-cell lymphoma	HR	high risk
DLCL	diffuse large-cell lymphoma	HRT	hormone replacement therapy
DTIC	dacarbazine	HSCT	hematopoietic stem-cell transplant
EBV	Epstein-Barr virus	IFN	interferon
ECOG	Eastern Cooperative Oncology Group	IL-2	interleukin-2
EFS	event-free survival	IMRT	intensity-modulated radiotherapy
EPO	epoetin alfa	IRB	institutional review board
FMEN	familial multiple endocrine neoplasia	IU	international units
FMTC	familial medullary thyroid carcinoma	LCIS	lobular cancer in situ
FNA	fine-needle aspiration	LVEF	left ventricular ejection fraction
5-FU	5-fluorouracil	LVSF	left ventricular shortening fraction
G-CSF	granulocyte colony–stimulating factor	Lx	lumpectomy
GM-CSF	granulocyte-macrophage colony–stimulating factor	m³	cubic meter
		mAb	monoclonal antibody
GPR	good partial remission	MBq	megabecquerel
GVHD	graft versus host disease	mcg	microgram
Gy	gray (unit of radiation)	mCi	millicurie
HCL	hairy cell leukemia	MDR	multidrug resistant
HD	Hodgkin's disease, high dose	MDS	myelodysplastic syndrome
HDC	high-dose chemotherapy	mets	metastases
		mg	milligram
HEPA	high-efficiency particulate air	mM	millimole
		mm	millimeter
HLA	human leukocyte antigens	6-MP	6-mercaptopurine
HNPCC	hereditary nonpolyposis colorectal cancer	MSDS	material safety data sheet

(continued)

MTD	maximum tolerated dose		PPE	personal protective equipment
MTX	methotrexate		PR	partial response, partial remission
MUD	matched unrelated donor		PSA	prostate-specific antigen
Mx	mastectomy		QALY	quality-adjusted life year
ng	nanogram		QoL	quality of life
NHL	non-Hodgkin's lymphoma		RCT	randomized clinical trial
NIOSH	National Institute for Occupational Safety and Health		REL	recommended exposure limit
NK	natural killer cells		RT	radiotherapy
NMSC	non-melanoma skin cancer		SAE	serious adverse event
NSCLC	non-small-cell lung cancer		SCC	squamous-cell carcinoma
OEL	occupational exposure limit		SCLC	small-cell lung cancer
OS	osteogenic sarcoma, overall survival		SD	stable disease
			SIADH	syndrome of inappropriate antidiuretic hormone secretion
OSHA	Occupational Safety and Health Administration		SWOG	Southwest Oncology Group
PBSC	peripheral blood stem cell		TBI	total body irradiation
PBSCH	peripheral blood stem-cell harvest		TCC	transitional-cell carcinoma
PBSCR	peripheral blood stem-cell rescue		TCP	thrombocytopenia
			6-TG	6-thioguanine
PBSCT	peripheral blood stem-cell transplant		TNF	tumor necrosis factor
			TNFa	tumor necrosis factor alpha
PD	progressive disease		TNM	tumor, nodes, metastasis
PEL	permissible exposure limit		TSG	tumor suppressor gene
			VNB	vinorelbine
PFS	progression-free survival		VP-16	etoposide

Normal laboratory values and calculations

Use the values and equations below as a quick-reference to both routine laboratory tests and oncology-related monitoring parameters. (Note: Reference values may differ somewhat among laboratories.)

Standard blood tests

Chemistry

Glucose
70 to 100 mg/dl

BUN
8 to 20 mg/dl

Creatinine
Men: 0.8 to 1.2 mg/dl
Women: 0.6 to 1.1 mg/dl

Sodium
135 to 145 mEq/L

Potassium
3.5 to 5 mEq/L

Anion gap
8 to 16 mEq/L

Chloride
100 to 108 mEq/L

Carbon dioxide
22 to 34 mEq/L

Albumin
3.3 to 4.5 g/dl

Calcium
9 to 10.5 mg/dl

Magnesium
1.5 to 2.5 mEq/L

Phosphorus
2.5 to 4.5 mg/dl

Protein
6 to 8.5 g/dl

Uric acid
Men: 4 to 8.5 mg/dl
Women: 2.5 to 7.5 mg/dl

Coagulation studies

Partial thromboplastin time
20 to 36 seconds

Prothrombin time
10 to 14 seconds

International Normalized Ratio (INR)
2 to 3 in patients receiving warfarin

Fibrinogen
215 to 519 mg/dl

Hematology

White blood cell count
4,100 to 10,900/mm^3

Red blood cell count
Men: 4.5 to 6.2 million/mm^3
Women: 4.2 to 5.4 million/mm^3

Hemoglobin
Men: 14 to 18 g/dl
Women: 12 to 16 g/dl

Hematocrit
Men: 42% to 54%
Women: 38% to 46%

Platelet count
40,000 to 400,000/mm^3

(continued)

Red blood cell indices
MCH: 26 to 32 pg
MCHC: 32 to 36 g/dl
MCV: 80 to 95 μm^3
White blood cell differential
Basophils: 0.3% to 2%
Eosinophils: 0.3% to 7%
Lymphocytes: 16.2% to 43%
Monocytes: 4% to 10%
Neutrophils: 47.6% to 76.8%

Iron studies

Serum iron
40 to 180 mcg/dl
Ferritin
Men: 18 to 270 ng/ml
Women: 18 to 160 ng/ml
Iron-binding capacity
200 to 450 mcg/dl
Transferrin
88 to 341 mg/dl
Transferrin saturation
12% to 57%

Lipids

Low-density lipoproteins
Optimal: < 100 mg/dl
Near optimal: 100 to 129 mg/dl
High-density lipoproteins
Desirable: ≥ 60 mg/dl
Total cholesterol
Desirable: < 200 mg/dl
Trigylcerides
Desirable: < 200 mg/dl

Liver function studies

Alanine aminotransferase
Men: 10 to 35 units/L
Women: 9 to 24 units/L
Alkaline phosphatase
39 to 117 units/L
Aspartate aminotransferase
Men: 8 to 20 units/L
Women: 5 to 40 units/L
Serum bilirubin
Direct: ≤ 0.4 mg/dl
Indirect: ≤ 1.3 mg/dl
Total: ≤ 1.3 mg/dl

Pancreatic enzymes

Amylase
30 to 170 U/L
Lipase
7 to 60 U/L

Thyroid studies

Triiodothyronine (T_3)
60 to 181 mg/dl
Thyroxine (T_4)
4.5 to 12.5 mcg/dl
Thyroid-stimulating hormone
0.5 to 4.5 mIU/L
Parathyroid hormone, intact
Ages 2 to 20: 9 to 52 pg/ml
Older than age 20: 8 to 97 pg/ml

Calculating creatinine clearance

Normal creatinine clearance ranges from 72 to 156 ml/minute/1.73 m^2. The three equations below are commonly used to calculate creatinine clearance.

Calculation using timed urine collection

Creatinine clearance (ml/minute) =

$$\frac{\text{urine creatinine (mg/dl)}}{\text{serum creatinine (mg/dl)}} \times \frac{\text{urine volume (ml)}}{\text{time*}}$$

(* Duration of urine collection: 1,440 minutes = 24 hours, 720 minutes = 12 hours, 480 minutes = 8 hours. Less than 20% variability with 8-, 12-, and 24-hour collection times.)

Estimating creatinine clearance using age, weight, and serum creatinine

Cockcroft-Gault method

Creatinine clearance$_{men}$ (ml/min) =

$$\frac{[(140 - \text{age}) \times (\text{lean body weight in kg})]}{72 \times \text{serum creatinine (mg/dl)}}$$

Creatinine clearance$_{women}$ (ml/min) =

$$0.85 \times \text{creatinine clearance}_{men}$$

Jelliffe method

This method assumes the patient has normal muscle mass and is used when urine cannot be collected.

Creatinine clearance (ml/min) =

$$98 - [0.8 \times (\text{age} - 20)]/\text{serum creatinine (mg/dl)}$$

(continued)

Calculating absolute neutrophil count

The absolute neutrophil count (ANC) is used to track a patient's response to chemotherapy and treatment for neutropenia. ANC should be above 1,500/mm^3. Here is a commonly used equation for calculating ANC:

$$ANC = \frac{WBCs \times (polymorphonuclear\ cells + bands)}{100}$$

Example:
WBC = 3,000 cells/mm^3
Polymorphonuclear cells = 60%
Bands = 3%

$$ANC = \frac{3,000 \times (60 + 3)}{100} = 3,000 \times 63 = 1,890\ cells/mm^3$$

Degrees of neutropenia
Mild: 1,000 to 1,500/mm^3
Moderate: 500 to 1,000/mm^3
Severe: < 500/mm^3

Calculating body surface area

Determining body surface area (BSA) is crucial to ensuring that patients receive optimal doses of chemotherapeutic drugs. The most commonly used formula for both adults and children is the Mosteller calculation.

Mosteller calculation

$$BSA\ (m^2) = \sqrt{\frac{height\ (cm) \times weight\ (kg)}{3,600}}$$

Average BSAs

Although BSA hinges largely on height and weight, age and gender also play a role, as the average BSAs below illustrate:

- Adult men: 1.9 m^2
- Adult women: 1.6 m^2
- Children ages 12 to 13: 1.33 m^2
- Children age 10: 1.14 m^2
- Children age 9: 1.07 m^2

Managing chemotherapy-induced nausea and vomiting

Chemotherapy-induced emesis can have an acute or delayed onset or can occur as breakthrough or anticipatory emesis. Use this guide to assess the emetogenic potential of chemotherapeutic drugs and choose appropriate antiemetic treatment.

Acute-onset emesis

Acute-onset emesis occurs within 24 hours after chemotherapy administration. Drugs that cause acute-onset emesis are divided into five levels. Level 5 drugs have the most emetogenic potential; level 1 drugs, the least.

When prescribing combination chemotherapy, determine emetogenic potential by identifying the most emetogenic drug in the combination and then assessing the emetic risk levels of the other drugs. A level 1 drug does not contribute to the combination's emetogenic level, whereas a drug from level 2, 3, or 4 increases emotogenic potential by one level greater than the most emetogenic drug in the combination. (For specific chemotherapy drugs associated with each risk level, see *Chemotherapy agents and emetic risk levels*, page 190.)

Level 5: High emetic risk (greater than 90% emesis frequency)
Start the following combination antiemetic regimen at least 30 minutes before each day's first chemotherapy dose:
- aprepitant 125 mg P.O. on day 1 only, followed by 80 mg P.O. daily on days 2 and 3
- dexamethasone 12 mg P.O. or I.V.
- *one* of the following 5-HT$_3$ antagonists:
   dolasetron 100 mg P.O. or 1.8 mg/kg I.V. or 100 mg I.V.
   granisetron 2 mg P.O. or 1 mg P.O. b.i.d. or 0.01 mg/kg I.V.
   ondansetron 16 to 24 mg P.O. or 8 to 12 mg (maximum, 32 mg) I.V.
   palonosetron 0.25 mg I.V. on day 1 only

Level 3 or 4: Moderate emetic risk (level 3—30% to 60% emesis frequency; level 4—60% to 90% emesis frequency)
Start the following combination antiemetic regimen at least 30 minutes before each day's first chemotherapy dose:
- dexamethasone 12 mg P.O. or I.V.

- *one* of the following 5-HT$_3$ antagonists:

  dolasetron 100 mg P.O. or 1.8 mg/kg I.V. or 100 mg I.V.

  granisetron 1 to 2 mg P.O. or 1 mg P.O. b.i.d. or 0.01 mg/kg (maximum, 1 mg) I.V.

  ondansetron 16 to 24 mg P.O. or 8 to 12 mg (maximum, 32 mg) I.V.

  palonosetron 0.25 mg I.V. on day 1 only

For patients receiving selected drugs in combination, consider aprepitant (125 mg P.O. on day 1 only, followed by 80 mg P.O. daily on days 2 and 3).

Level 2: Low emetic risk (10% to 30% emesis frequency)

Start the following single-agent antiemetic regimen at least 30 minutes before each day's first chemotherapy dose:

- dexamethasone 12 mg P.O. or I.V.; or prochlorperazine 10 mg P.O. or I.V. every 4 to 6 hours or 15 mg spansule P.O. every 8 to 12 hours; or metoclopramide 20 to 40 mg P.O. every 4 to 6 hours or 1 to 2 mg/kg I.V. every 3 to 4 hours and diphenhydramine 25 to 50 mg P.O. or I.V. every 4 to 6 hours

Level 1: Minimal emetic risk (less than 10% emesis frequency)

No routine emesis prophylaxis is required. If the patient experiences nausea and vomiting at any time up to 24 hours after the first chemotherapy dose, consider using the regimen recommended for low emetic risk.

Delayed-onset emesis

Delayed-onset emesis occurs after the first 24 hours of chemotherapy administration. Continue recommended antiemetic therapy for at least 4 days before adding a delayed-onset regimen, except in patients receiving palonosetron, which is given only on day 1 of therapy.

For patients receiving high-emetic-risk chemotherapy drugs, add one of the following to the regimen:

- dexamethasone 8 mg P.O. or I.V. daily or 4 mg P.O. or I.V. b.i.d.
- metoclopramide 20 to 40 mg P.O. or I.V. every 6 hours and diphenhydramine 25 to 50 mg P.O. or I.V. every 4 to 6 hours as needed, plus dexamethasone 8 mg P.O. or I.V. daily or 4 mg P.O. or I.V. b.i.d.

In addition to either regimen above, add one of the following 5-HT$_3$ antagonists:

- dolasetron 100 mg P.O. daily or 1.8 mg/kg I.V. or 100 mg I.V.

- granisetron 1 to 2 mg P.O. daily or 1 mg P.O. b.i.d. or 0.01 mg/kg (maximum, 1 mg) I.V.
- ondansetron 8 mg P.O. twice daily, or 16 mg P.O. daily or 8 mg I.V.

For patients receiving cisplatin, dexamethasone with metoclopramide or a 5-HT$_3$ antagonist alone is recommended.

For patients receiving low- to intermediate-emetic-risk drugs, no regular antiemetic prophylaxis is recommended for delayed-onset emesis.

Breakthrough emesis

Breakthrough emesis occurs during the course of chemotherapy when an antiemetic regimen is not effective. If the patient has nausea and vomiting, add *one* of the following antiemetic regimens to the acute-onset regimen:

- dexamethasone 12 mg P.O. or I.V. daily (if not given previously)
- dolasetron 100 mg P.O. daily or 1.8 mg/kg I.V. or 100 mg I.V.
- granisetron 1 to 2 mg P.O. once daily or 1 mg P.O. twice daily or 0.01 mg/kg (maximum, 1 mg) I.V.
- haloperidol 1 to 2 mg P.O. every 4 to 6 hours or 1 to 3 mg I.V. every 4 to 6 hours
- lorazepam 0.5 to 2 mg P.O. every 4 to 6 hours
- metoclopramide 20 to 40 mg P.O. every 4 to 6 hours as needed or 1 to 2 mg/kg I.V. every 3 to 4 hours, plus diphenhydramine 25 to 50 mg P.O. or I.V. every 4 to 6 hours
- olanzapine 2.5 to 5 mg P.O. twice daily as needed
- ondansetron 8 mg P.O. or I.V. daily
- prochlorperazine 10 mg P.O. every 4 to 6 hours or 25 mg P.R. every 12 hours or spansules 15 mg P.O. every 8 to 12 hours
- promethazine 25 to 50 mg P.O. or P.R. every 6 hours as needed

Anticipatory emesis

Anticipatory emesis occurs before chemotherapy begins. Add *one* of the following single-agent antiemetic regimens, starting the night before chemotherapy:

- alprazolam 0.5 mg P.O. three times daily
- lorazepam 0.5 to 2 mg P.O., I.V., or sublingually every 6 hours

Chemotherapy agents and emetic risk levels

Level 5: High emetic risk
Emesis frequency: More than 90%

Chemotherapy agent

altretamine
carmustine > 250 mg/m^2
cisplatin ≥ 50 mg/m^2
cyclophosphamide > 1,500 mg/m^2
dacarbazine

doxorubicin or epirubicin
   with cyclophosphamide
lomustine > 60 mg/m^2
mechorethamine
streptozocin

Level 4: Moderate emetic risk
Emesis frequency: 60% to 90%

Chemotherapy agent

amifostine > 500 mg/m^2
busulfan > 4 mg daily
carboplatin
carmustine ≤ 250 mg/m^2
cisplatin < 50 mg/m^2
cyclophosphamide > 750 mg/m^2
   to ≤ 1,500 mg/m^2

cytarabine (except in low
   doses)
dactinomycin
doxorubicin ≥ 60 mg/m^2
epirubicin > 90 mg/m^2
melphalan > 50 mg/m^2
methotrexate > 1,000 mg/m^2
procarbazine (oral)

Level 3: Moderate emetic risk
Emesis frequency: 30% to 60%

Chemotherapy agent

aldesleukin
amifostine > 300 to ≤ 500 mg/m^2
arsenic trioxide
cyclophosphamide ≤ 750 mg/m^2
cyclophosphamide (oral)
daunorubicin
doxorubicin 20 to < 60 mg/m^2
doxorubicin liposomal
epirubicin ≤ 90 mg/m^2
hexamethylmelamine (oral)

idarubicin
ifosfamide
interleukin-2 > 12 to 15 million units/m^2
irinotecan
lomustine < 60 mg/m^2
methotrexate 250 to 1,000
   mg/m^2
mitoxantrone < 15 mg/m^2
oxaliplatin > 75 mg/m^2

Level 2: Low emetic risk
Emesis frequency: 10% to 30%

Chemotherapy agent
amifostine ≤ 300 mg
asparaginase
bexarotene
bortezomib
cytarabine 100 to 200 mg/m^2
capecitabine
docetaxel
doxorubicin < 20 mg/m^2
etoposide
fludarabine
fluorouracil
gemcitabine

mercaptopurine
methotrexate > 50 to < 250 mg/m^2
mitomycin
paclitaxel
pemetrexed
temozolomide
teniposide
thiotepa
trimetrexate
topotecan

Level 1: Minimal emetic risk
Emesis frequency: Less than 10%

Chemotherapy agent
alemtuzumab
asparaginase
azacitidine
bevacizumab
bleomycin
bortezomib
busulfan
cetuximab
chlorambucil (oral)
cladribine
denileukin diftitox
dexrazoxane
erlotinib
estramustine
fludarabine
gefitinib
gemtuzumab ozogamicin
hormones

hydroxyurea
imatinib mesylate
interferon alfa
melphalan (oral low dose)
methotrexate ≤ 50 mg/m^2
mitotane
pegaspargase
pentostatin
rituximab
thioguanine (oral)
tositumomab
trastuzumab
uracil
valrubicin
vinblastine
vincristine
vinorelbine

Managing anemia

Anemia occurs in nearly half of cancer patients even before treatment begins. Once chemotherapy starts, anemia is a near certainty. Anemia and the associated fatigue are more than a quality-of-life issue; they can significantly affect patient outcome as well.

Treatment

The guidelines below focus on cancer- or treatment-related anemia.

If the patient is asymptomatic but has risk factors for anemia:
• Observe the patient, and consider erythropoietic therapy.
• If erythropoietic therapy is being considered, obtain iron studies and prescribe iron supplements as indicated. Typically, such supplements are indicated by a ferritin level below 100 mcg/ml or transferrin saturation below 20%. Titrate dosages to maintain an optimal hemoglobin value (12 g/dl).
• If hemoglobin is 12 g/dl, or more than 2 g/dl lower than the initial level, and symptoms have not improved, consider erythropoietic therapy. If hemoglobin is 12 g/dl, or more than 2 g/dl lower than the initial level, and symptoms have improved, titrate the dosage of the erythropoietic agent or iron preparation to maintain a hemoglobin level of at least 12 g/dl.

If the patient is symptomatic:
• Transfuse appropriate blood products. If hemoglobin is 10 to 11 g/dl, consider erythropoietic therapy; if hemoglobin is below 10 g/dl, strongly consider erythropoietic therapy.
• Obtain iron studies and administer iron supplements as indicated (for ferritin level below 100 mcg/ml or transferrin saturation below 20%). Titrate dosage to maintain optimal hemoglobin (12 g/dl).
• Reevaluate symptoms and hemoglobin at each follow-up visit.
• If hemoglobin is 12 g/dl, or more than 2 g/dl lower than the initial level, and symptoms have improved, titrate the dosage of the erythropoietic agent or iron preparation to maintain a hemoglobin level of at least 12 g/dl.

Managing febrile neutropenia

Neutropenia increases a cancer patient's mortality risk, lengthens hospitalization, and increases medical costs. In many cases, fever is the first—and sometimes only—sign of neutropenia.

Treatment

Choose therapy based on risk assessment findings, the patient's condition, clinical evaluation, infection site, and previous antibiotic therapy. Optimally, treatment should start within the first few hours of clinical presentation of signs and symptoms, with follow-up as needed.

Initial therapy

Initial therapy for neutropenia may involve oral combination therapy, I.V. monotherapy, or I.V. dual therapy. Vancomycin therapy is usually avoided due to the emergence of vancomyin-resistant organisms.

Oral combination therapy is used for low-risk adults only. Typically, it involves ciprofloxacin and amoxicillin/clavulanate. In patients with penicillin allergy, substitute clindamycin for amoxicillin/clavulanate.

For *I.V. monotherapy,* choose one of the following:
- carbapenem
- cefepime (check susceptibility for local antibiogram)
- ceftazidime (provides weak gram-positive coverage, is associated with increased breakthrough infections)
- imipenem and cilastatin
- meropenem
- piperacillin and tazobactam (may interfere with galactomannan measurement).

For *I.V. dual therapy,* choose one of these regimens:
- an aminoglycoside and an antipseudomonal penicillin or extended-spectrum cephalosporin (such as cefepime or ceftazidime), with or without a beta-lactamase inhibitor; or an aminoglycoside with an extended-spectrum cephalosporin (such as cefepime or ceftazidime)
- ciprofloxacin and an antipseudomonal penicillin.

Managing diarrhea

Diarrhea can decrease the patient's quality of life and seriously jeopardize outcome. Based on severity of symptoms, NCI grades diarrhea on a scale from 1 (mild) to 4 (severe or life-threatening).

Treatment guide

Treatment of diarrhea takes a stepped approach and varies according to NCI grade. For patients with grade 2 diarrhea, withhold cytotoxic chemotherapy until symptoms abate, and consider reducing the dosage of chemotherapy.

Initial treatment

• Administer loperamide 4 mg P.O. initially, then 2 mg every 4 hours or after every unformed stool. Do not exceed 16 mg daily. Discontinue loperamide when the patient has been diarrhea-free for 12 hours.

Continued treatment (NCI grade 1 or 2)

• Administer loperamide 2 mg P.O. every 2 hours until the patient has been diarrhea-free for 12 hours. Patients may take 4 mg every 4 hours during the night.
• Administer oral antibiotics.
• If the patient progresses to NCI grade 3 or 4, treat as described below for severe diarrhea.

Treatment of persistent diarrhea (NCI grade 1 or 2)

• Evaluate stool specimens, CBC, and electrolytes.
• Replace electrolytes as needed.
• Discontinue loperamide and start second-line treatment—octreotide 100 to 150 mcg subcutaneously three times daily, up to 500 mcg three times daily; or tincture of opium 0.6 ml P.O. four times daily.

Treatment of severe diarrhea (NCI grade 3 or 4)

• Admit the patient to the hospital.
• Administer octreotide 100 to 150 mcg subcutaneously three times daily. As needed, titrate up to 500 mcg three times daily based on response, or administer 25 to 50 mcg/hour by continuous I.V. infusion.
• Administer I.V. fluids and antibiotics as needed.
• Discontinue cytotoxic chemotherapy until symptoms resolve; then restart at reduced dosage.

Managing oral mucositis

Mucositis affects approximately 40% of cancer patients. It is a major concern because it can lead to such life-threatening conditions as sepsis, infection, and malnutrition.

Treatment

Examine the patient's oral mucosa daily, and teach the patient how to perform this examination at home. Additional recommendations include the following:

• Advise the patient to use bland mouth rinses, such as normal saline solution and sodium bicarbonate.

• If sores crust over, instruct the patient to rinse with equal parts hydrogen peroxide and water or salt water (1 tsp salt in 4 cups water) for no more than 2 days. (A longer period impedes healing.)

• Instruct the patient to use a soft, nylon-bristled toothbrush and to avoid dental floss and water-pressure gum cleaners.

• As indicated, prescribe mucosal-coating agents (such as antacid solutions, kaolin solutions, and Amphojel), water-soluble lubricating agents (including artificial saliva for xerostomia), or topical anesthetics (such as 2% viscous lidocaine or benzocaine spray or gel). Instruct the patient to rinse or irrigate the mouth before using these agents, to remove particles and debris.

• Culture mucosal lesions. Candidal lesions appear as whitish plaque.

• Use cryotherapy to cool the oral cavity and help prevent oral mucositis. Cooling causes vasoconstriction, which seems to limit absorption of mucotoxic agents by the oral mucosa.

• For oral bleeding, instruct the patient to rinse the mouth with a mixture of one part 3% hydrogen peroxide to two or three parts saltwater solution (1 tsp salt in 4 cups water) to help clean the wound. Stress the importance of rinsing carefully so as not to disturb clots.

• Instruct the patient to avoid irritating agents, such as commercial mouthwashes containing phenol, astringents, or alcohol, as well as lemon-glycerin swabs and solutions. Also discourage tobacco use and alcohol consumption.

Managing hazardous drugs

For the past decade, concern about the safety of health care workers who handle hazardous drugs has been growing. Up to 5.5 million health care workers have the potential to be exposed to hazardous drugs. Anyone involved in caring for patients receiving such drugs may be vulnerable. Generally, the activities that pose the greatest risk to health care workers are preparing and administering cancer chemotherapy agents, cleaning up chemotherapy spills, and handling patient excreta.

Hazardous drugs are toxic compounds that meet one or more of the following criteria:
- carcinogenic
- genotoxic (mutagenic)
- teratogenic (developmentally toxic)
- toxic to human reproductive capability
- organotoxic in humans or animals when given in low doses
- new drugs that mimic existing hazardous drugs in structure or toxicity.

Also, on direct contact, these agents may irritate the skin, eyes, and mucous membranes and cause ulceration and tissue necrosis.

Many hazardous drugs used in cancer treatment bind to or damage DNA. Other antineoplastics, some antivirals, antibiotics, and bioengineered drugs interfere with cell growth or proliferation or with DNA synthesis.

Preparing and administering parenteral drugs

Wear gloves, a gown, and a face shield (if necessary) when preparing, handling, and administering hazardous parenteral drugs. Use stringent aseptic technique during any procedure in which sterile dosage forms are manipulated with needles and syringes. Needleless devices reduce the risk of blood-borne pathogen exposure and accidental exposure to hazardous drugs caused by needlesticks.

Drug reconstitution, withdrawal, and transfer

When reconstituting a hazardous drug in a vial, avoid pressurizing the vial contents, which may cause the drug to spray out around the needle or through a needle hole or a loose seal. To avoid pressurization, create a *slight* negative pressure in the vial. After drawing up the diluent, insert the needle into the vial and pull back the plunger; this action creates a slight negative pressure inside the vial, which draws air into the syringe. Transfer small amounts of diluent slowly as equal volumes of air are removed.

Keeping the needle in the vial, swirl the contents carefully until they dissolve. With the vial inverted, gradually withdraw the proper amount of drug solution while equal volumes of air are exchanged for solution. Measure the exact volume needed while the needle is in the vial; any excess drug should remain in the vial. With the vial upright, withdraw the plunger past the original starting point to create a slight negative pressure before removing the needle. Make sure the needle hub is clear before you remove the needle.

To withdraw a hazardous drug from an ampule, gently tap the neck or top portion of the ampule. Then wipe the neck with alcohol and attach a 5-micron filter needle or straw to a syringe large enough so that it is no more than three-quarters full when holding the drug. Next, draw the fluid through the filter needle or straw and clear it from the needle and hub. Exchange the needle or straw for a needle of similar gauge and length; eject any air and excess drug into a sterile vial (leaving the desired volume in the syringe), taking care to avoid aerosolization.

If the dose will be dispensed in the syringe, draw back the plunger to clear fluid from the needle and hub. Replace the needle with a locking cap, and surface-decontaminate and label the syringe. Use a syringe that is no more than three-quarters full when filled with the solution; this reduces the risk of the plunger separating from the syringe barrel.

When transferring a hazardous drug to an I.V. bag, take care to puncture only the septum of the injection port—not the sides of the port or the bag. After the drug solution has been injected into the I.V. bag, surface-decontaminate the I.V. port, container, and set. Label the final preparation and cover the injection port with a protective shield.

General recommendations

General recommendations for preparing and administering hazardous parenteral drugs include the following:
- Always work below eye level.
- Visually examine the drug dose while it is still in the transport bag. If the dose appears to be intact, remove it from the bag.

• Place a plastic-backed absorbent pad under the drug administration area to absorb leaks and prevent drug contact with the patient's skin.

• Whenever possible, use a needleless system to administer a hazardous I.V. drug, with Luer-Lok fittings for the system itself, syringes, needles, infusion tubing, and pumps. Place gauze pads under the connection at injection ports to catch leaks, and keep a spill kit and hazardous drug waste container readily available.

• Prime the I.V. tubing (if required) with a solution that does not contain hazardous drugs. or use the backflow method.

• To administer hazardous I.M. or subcutaneous drugs, use Luer-Lok safety needles or retracting needles or shields. Make sure syringes have Luer-locking connections and are less than three-quarters full. Keep a spill kit and hazardous drug waste container readily available. Remove the syringe cap and connect the appropriate safety needle. Do not expel air from the syringe or prime the safety needle. After administration, discard the syringe, with safety needle attached, directly into a hazardous drug waste container.

• Discard hazardous drug containers with the administration sets attached; do not remove the sets.

• Use a transport bag as a containment bag for materials contaminated with hazardous drugs, drug containers, and sets.

• Use detergent, sodium hypochlorite solution, and neutralizer (if appropriate) to wash surfaces that may have come in contact with hazardous drugs.

• Wearing gloves, contain and dispose of materials contaminated with hazardous drugs and remaining personal protective equipment (PPE) as hazardous waste. Make sure the hazardous drug waste container is large enough to hold all the discarded material and PPE. Do not push or force contaminated materials into the container.

• After disposing of materials, carefully remove, contain, and discard your gloves. Then wash your hands thoroughly.

Preparing and administering oral and noninjectable drugs

Oral forms of certain hazardous drugs may be prescribed for small children or for adults with feeding tubes. Recipes for extemporaneously compounded oral liquids may start with the parenteral form or may require crushing of tablets or opening of capsules, which may cause fine dust formation and local environmental contamination. Also, tablets or capsules may be coated with a dust of residual hazardous drug that could be inhaled, absorbed through the skin, or ingested or could spread to other locations. Also, liquid formulations may be aerosolized or spilled.

General recommendations

General recommendations for preparing and administering hazardous oral or noninjectable drugs include the following:

• Work below eye level during drug preparation.
• Never crush or compound a hazardous oral drug in an unprotected environment.
• Visually examine the drug dose while it is still in the transport bag. If it appears to be intact, remove it from the transport bag.
• Keep a spill kit and hazardous drug waste container readily available.
• Wash hands and don double gloves. Wear a face shield if the potential for sprays, aerosols, or splashing exists.
• Place a plastic-backed absorbent pad on the work area, if necessary, to contain spills.
• After administration, contain and dispose of contaminated materials into a hazardous drug waste container. Do not push or force contaminated materials into the container.
• Carefully remove, contain, and discard your gloves. Wash your hands thoroughly.

Dealing with accidental exposure

In case of skin contact with a cytotoxic drug, immediately remove contaminated clothing and wash the affected area thoroughly with soap and water. (Do not use a scrub brush because this could abrade the skin.) Rinse the area thoroughly. Call for help, if needed. Then obtain medical attention.

In case of eye contact, flush the affected eye (while holding back the eyelid) with copious amounts of water or normal saline solution for at least 15 minutes. Call for help, if needed. Then obtain medical attention.

Index